Vitamin B12 and Folic Acid

by Ruth Adams
and
Frank Murray

Larchmont Books
New York

NOTICE: This book is meant as an informational guide for the prevention of disease. For conditions of ill-health, we recommend that you see a physician, psychiatrist or other professional licensed to treat disease. These days, many medical practitioners are discovering that a strong nutritional program supports and fortifies whatever therapy they may use, as well as effectively preventing a recurrence of the illness.

Second Printing: January, 1983
First Printing: March, 1981

VITAMIN B12 AND FOLIC ACID

ISBN 0-915962-31-4

Printed in the United States of America

LARCHMONT BOOKS
6 East 43rd Street
New York, N.Y. 10017
Tel., 212-949-0800

Contents

CHAPTER 1

Your Need for Vitamin B_{12} and Folic Acid

WE USUALLY THINK of anemia having to do with lack of iron in food, and doctors often tell patients that they have iron deficiency anemia. However, there are other types of anemia, i.e., pernicious anemia and macrocytic anemia, both of which are respectively due to a deficiency in vitamin B_{12} and folic acid, another B vitamin. As you will see throughout this book, these two water-soluble B vitamins are closely related in the body, hence the reason we are discussing them in one book. There are other forms of anemia, such as that caused by a vitamin B_2 (riboflavin) deficiency, but, for the purposes of this book, we are confining most of our discussions about anemia to vitamin B_{12} and folic acid.

Naturally, there are other conditions of ill health which may be prevented by these two vitamins other than anemia. We go into these conditions in greater detail in later chapters, such as prevention of certain skin conditions like psoriasis; mental illness; protection from The Pill; the importance of these two vitamins during pregnancy; Crohn's Disease; certain kinds of cancer; etc. And we explain why some vegetarians, senior citizens and pregnant women may be short on these two B vitamins, especially vitamin B_{12}.

Folic acid—sometimes referred to in the medical literature as folacin and pteroylmonoglutamic acid—is essential for forming certain body proteins. It is important for maintaining certain functions in the intestinal tract, and, as previously reported, it prevents macrocytic anemia, which causes blood cells to become unusually large.

Symptoms of folic acid deficiency include: weakness and loss of appetite and energy; digestive complaints; anemia resembling pernicious anemia; diarrhea; lack of ability to absorb food; and inflammation of the tongue.

Vitamin B_{12}—occasionally called cobalamin or cyanocobalamin—is the substance which prevents pernicious anemia. Lack of this vitamin causes progressive involvement of the nerves which eventually reaches the spinal cord. Untreated, it can be fatal. Pernicious anemia depletes the body's store of iron and contributes to a degeneration of all body cells, especially those in the intestines, nervous system and bone marrow. As might be expected, this B vitamin is necessary to synthesize hemoglobin and to help manufacture healthy red blood cells.

Chromosomes are microscopic parts of cells which contain the genes by which heredity is determined. Damage to chromosomes has become one symptom by which doctors can diagnose certain diseases, such as mongolism. Now we have evidence from a Public Health Service physician specializing in leukemia that vitamins can repair chromosome damage.

Dr. Clark W. Heath reported in the magazine *Blood* that vitamin B_{12} and folic acid are involved in certain functions that go on in chromosomes, and lack of these vitamins may result in damage to the chromosomes. Fifteen patients were studied. Both blood and bone marrow cells showed damage to the chromosomes. After treatment with vitamin B_{12}, folic acid, or both, the chromosomes returned to normal.

A certain kind of anemia produced the most striking changes. Dr. Heath went on to say that a wide variety of medical findings are encountered in patients with deficiencies with vitamin B_{12} and folic acid. The only reliable source of vitamin B_{12} in everyday meals is liver, which is also an excellent source of folic acid.

"The majority of women taking oral contraceptives (The Pill) have been shown to have abnormal tryptophan (an amino acid) metabolism, indicating a relative vitamin B_6 (pyridoxine) deficiency, and some of these have evidence of absolute deficiency of this vitamin. These abnormalities are abolished by the administration of 20 to 30 milligrams of vitamin B_6 daily, which is some 10 times the usual intake," according to Victor Wynn, Laboratory for Metabolic Research, St. Mary's Hospital, London, England, as reported by Hoffmann-LaRoche, Inc., Nutley, New Jersey.

Similarly, the drug company reported, people with lowered levels of folic acid and vitamin B_{12}—often associated with oral contraceptive use—have been shown to respond to vitamin therapy. In a study of 176 women on The Pill and 140 controls, Dr. A. M. Shojania, Associate Professor of Pediatrics, University of Manitoba, Canada, showed that women on the pill had significantly lower serum and red-cell folate and higher urinary excretion of folic acid than did the controls. They later showed that serum-folic acid levels in oral contraceptive users fell with duration of use. The percentage of subjects with pathologically low serum-folate levels rose progressively with oral contraceptive use from nine per cent during the first year to 21 per cent at two years and 42 per cent after four years. Only two per cent of their control subjects had pathologically low folate levels. Dr. Shojania later stated that, "The review of the literature leaves no doubt that oral contraceptives interfere with folate metabolism."

The New Jersey vitamin company also discussed the work of Dr. Richard R. Streiff, Chief Medical Services, Veterans

Administration Hospital, Gainesville, Fla., whose tests suggest that orally administered contraceptives can have an adverse effect in some women on the absorption of dietary folate. In his study, seven women aged 21 to 39 with folic acid deficiency and anemia were treated at the University of Florida. One of the patients did not respond to dietary folic acid, but went through rapid remission when oral supplements of folic acid were given. Four other patients responded in a similar fashion.

In reviewing 47 subsequent similar cases, which he analyzed in the *Journal of the American Medical Association*, Dr. Streiff said that "Folate deficiency associated with oral administration of contraceptives does not necessarily require discontinuance of the drug regimen but folic acid therapy is definitely indicated."

For the record, women on The Pill may also have vitamin C deficiencies, Hoffmann-LaRoche stated. For example, Drs. J. M. Rivers and M. M. Devine, professors of Nutritional Science, Cornell University, have reported that the lowest levels of vitamin C appear after extended oral contraceptive use. In their study, two women not taking The Pill and four women using oral contraceptives were studied. The latter tended to show maximum vitamin C levels when they were off the pill. Oral load tests showed that the tablets did not cause increased urinary excretion of the vitamin C.

And Drs. M. A. Briggs and M. I. Briggs of Alfred Hospital, Melbourne, Australia, have demonstrated that the estrogen component of The Pill lowers tissue levels of vitamin C. They added that women taking oral contraceptives are often deficient in vitamin C, vitamin B_2, vitamin B_6, vitamin B_{12} and vitamin E. They recommend daily vitamin supplements for most women using The Pill.

A letter to the editor of *The Lancet*, October 9, 1965, states that all psychiatric patients should be tested for vitamin B_{12} deficiency, before treatment is decided upon. Two groups of people especially susceptible to this deficiency are those who have had surgery of the digestive tract and those who have been treated with certain drugs.

It is possible, says this expert, that patients may have none of the classic signs of anemia, yet still be deficient enough in vitamin B_{12} to have symptoms of mental illness. It is, of course, possible to be deficient in vitamin B_{12} simply because you do not eat foods that contain it.

Glaucoma is a serious eye condition which, if left untreated, may result in blindness. It is caused by the retention of fluids within the cavity of the eye, which exert pressure on the delicate lining. Russian researchers reported in 1961 and 1963 on treating this condition by injecting vitamin B_{12}. They gave a daily dose of one-tenth of a milligram to 46 patients and obtained improvement in about half of the patients.

A Japanese physician has confirmed their findings by giving one milligram of vitamin B_{12} injected twice a week for one month. The sight of seven of the affected 17 eyes improved, 10 gained in their field of vision, 10 showed a drop in pressure in the eye, and 13 improved in other ways. This is apparently an example of how a vitamin can be used as a drug, for there is no indication that glaucoma is caused by lack of vitamin B_{12} in the diet. Since the treatment is harmless and inexpensive, we wish American physicians would try it. The report we read appears in *New Scientist*, a British publication, for August 13, 1964.

Many of the women who long for children without being able to conceive may be suffering from lack of vitamin B_{12}. Researchers at the Royal Infirmary in Glasgow, Scotland have found that women who could not have children for many years became pregnant when pernicious anemia was diagnosed and they were given injections of B_{12}.

One woman, for example, married at 25, remained childless for 11 years and no cause could be found for her infertility. Then she developed the symptoms of pernicious anemia—fatigue and a tingling in the hands and feet. She was given vitamin B_{12} therapy and became pregnant 11 months later.

If ordinary anemia, caused by lack of iron, were responsible for infertility, say the doctors, 10 per cent of all women would be unable to have children since that many suffer from iron deficiency anemia. But pernicious anemia is much more difficult to diagnose, so it goes undiscovered for years until the telltale symptoms of an advanced case appear.

The Journal of the American Medical Association reported in June, 1956 on the work of Dr. I. S. Klemes who used vitamin B_{12} against bursitis. This physician used injections of vitamin B_{12}—daily doses of 1,000 micrograms (not milligrams) of the vitamin injected not into the painful joint, but anywhere the doctor decides to inject it.

After a week of these daily injections, they are continued three times a week for two or three weeks, then once a week for two or three weeks or until the pain disappears. We have heard from many acquaintances that this therapy worked for them, although they had not had success in treating their bursitis by taking vitamin B_{12} by mouth.

In older folks especially, injections of this vitamin appear to be astonishingly successful in preventing and treating a variety of ailments, although taking this vitamin by mouth cannot achieve the same results. The reason is probably that the older digestive tract lacks enough of a substance which is essential for absorbing the vitamin. It's called "Intrinsic substance." Then, too, it's hard to get enough of vitamin B_{12} to achieve near miracles of healing if you are taking it by mouth. But an injection of as much as 1,000 micrograms is painless, harmless and, apparently, very effective.

Chloromycetin is an antibiotic with a considerable potential for harm if it is used in the wrong way, given in excessive doses or for prolonged periods to susceptible people. Hundreds of cases have been reported in medical literature in which the patients suffered anything from mild symptoms to death after taking this drug. Most commonly, the blood forming organs in the bone marrow were affected so that the patient suffered from a certain deadly kind of anemia.

The American Journal of Diseases of Children, October, 1967, reports on the case of a 12-year-old child with cystic fibrosis who was given this drug and developed optic neuritis as a side effect. This is inflammation of the nerves of the eye, resulting in pain and difficulty in seeing. Each time she was given the antibiotic, the neuritis appeared.

Then her doctors gave her large doses of vitamin B_{12} and vitamin B_6, along with the antibiotic. There was no recurrence of the neuritis. And doses of the antibiotic given with the vitamins were considerably larger than the earlier doses had been. Presumably the child continued to take the drug to combat the infection which she had, and will suffer no harm from it so long as the very large doses of B vitamins are given along with it.

It may take years before laboratory chemists discover just how the B vitamins act to protect against this drug. And when the discovery comes, it will involve something very complex and probably incomprehensible to the non-scientist. But surely all of us can understand and profit by the knowledge that the B vitamins are powerful forces for good. Who knows what other antibiotics may be doing us harm which could be prevented by massive doses of the B vitamins? What harm would it do to experiment a bit more along these lines rather than just giving another drug to counteract the bad effects of the first drug?

Deficiency in vitamin B_{12} is directly responsible for certain nerve disorders which may produce unpleasant or painful symptoms, especially in arms, legs or feet. In the October, 1965 issue of *Archives of Neurology*, Dr. R. F. Mayer describes patients who had past or present deficiency in vitamin

B_{12} to whom he gave tests for nerve function. At the same time he tested other patients who did not have this deficiency.

He found that the farthest ends of the nerves may be affected by the vitamin B_{12} deficiency, although the nearer portion of the nerve remains healthy. In a few patients the nerve function returned to normal when they took vitamin B_{12} for six to 12 months.

It is well known that pernicious anemia responds well to treatment with vitamin B_{12}. And it is known that patients with this kind of anemia suffer from nerve damage, sometimes severe enough to cause death. Says the *Journal of the American Medical Association* for October 11, 1965, commenting on Dr. Mayer's findings, "Although vitamin B_{12} deficiency is now well recognized and both the hematological and neurological (blood and nerve) symptoms respond to treatment with cyanocobalamin, patients with this deficiency are still common."

This gives you some idea of how important vitamin B_{12} and folic acid are in maintaining good health. Now let's look at other ways in which these two important B vitamins work together and separately to keep us healthy.

CHAPTER 2

Conquering the Plague That Was Pernicious Anemia

In 1934 three American physicians received the Nobel prize for their work in establishing the cause and cure of pernicious anemia. In these days of highly sophisticated laboratory procedures and many kinds of gadgetry for testing and treating patients, the story of those early days makes fascinating reading. Most doctors in those days were dedicated people who sometimes risked their own and their patient's lives and their future careers when they took chances with curing a fatal disease like pernicious anemia with a simple food substance—liver.

For that's what the cure finally consisted of. In *Medical World News* for September 8, 1972, Dr. William P. Murphy, one of the Nobel winners, tells the story of his work on pernicious anemia and his discovery that liver would cure it. Dr. Murphy is now 80 years old. He still practices medicine in Massachusetts.

He was a specialist in the study of blood at Peter Bent Brigham Hospital in Boston during the early days of blood transfusion, the 1920's. There was no treatment for victims of pernicious anemia. When their red blood count went down below a certain level, they died, unless they could be given blood transfusions. There were no blood banks, no way to store blood. It was taken directly from the donor, into a flask containing an anticoagulant, then injected immediately into the arm of the patient. Sometimes patients needed as many as 100 transfusions. Nothing was known of blood types except for a knowledge of Type A, B, AB and O. In spite of this, says Dr. Murphy, there were no serious reactions. One night a patient of Dr. Murphy's appeared doomed to die of pernicious anemia by the next morning. Dr. Murphy went to his house and gave him a transfusion of his own blood.

Meanwhile, a University of Rochester physician Dr. George H. Whipple reported he had found that liver, given to anemic dogs, appeared to cure them almost miraculously. Although pernicious anemia was obviously not the same thing as iron deficiency anemia, Dr. Murphy decided to try it. He decided to run a test at the hospital, giving each patient one-fourth to one-half pound of liver daily.

He had difficulty with the administration of the hospital which was not a bit interested in doing research, but simply wanted to be sure that no patient's life was endangered. Would Dr. Murphy guarantee that no patient's life would be endangered? he was asked. If the liver diet failed, would he surely agree to give transfusions, even though this was bound to interfere with the results he was trying to show? Blood transfusions were a novelty in those days and the staff wanted experience in giving them!

He finally had permission and started to feed a patient on liver. The man was in a coma with a red cell blood count of only 800,000—a dangerously low level. Dr. Murphy had found that it usually took about five days for the liver therapy to increase the numbers of red blood cells. This patient had shown no improvement by the fifth day. It was time to give him a transfusion which would bring the blood count up again and hide the effects of the liver treatment. Dr. Murphy noticed that there was just a tiny increase in the blood cell count and he decided to wait until morning for the transfusion. He spent a sleepless night, he tells us, and returned fearfully to find the patient sitting up in bed demanding his breakfast. The impossible had happened. The half-pound of liver daily for five days had worked the miracle. This patient survived and lived for many more years, Dr. Murphy tells us.

That year Dr. Murphy treated 45 pernicious anemia patients with liver every day and had no failures. It wasn't easy. Some of the patients didn't like liver. Sometimes the liver was tough. They did not dare to cook it with onions or bacon for fear these might interfere with the experiment in some way. Sometimes they gave raw liver finely ground. Sometimes they fed it by stomach tube.

In 1926 Dr. Murphy published his first paper on liver therapy for pernicious anemia in the *Journal of the American Medical Association*. The next year he treated 60 patients successfully. And doctors all over the country began to use this treatment and report success. Some of these had been trying other diet experiments—high fat diet, high protein diets and so on.

Now it was necessary to make an extract of the liver, if possible, so that it could be given in concentrated form and the patient would not have to choke down liver at two meals every day. Dr. Murphy and several other researchers worked on this problem and solved it. They produced a liver extract which contained the substance (whatever it was) that cured pernicious anemia. They made it in such purified form that it could even be injected without severe side effects.

By 1946 other researchers announced they had identified the mysterious but potent substance in liver which cures pernicious anemia. It was folic acid, they said, a vitamin of the B group. This was accepted for treatment and used. But somehow things didn't work out. Most symptoms of pernicious anemia were cured by folic acid, but patients still had the nervous symptoms of pernicious anemia which were very serious, involving difficulty in walking, "pins and needles" in arms and legs, even psychotic behavior, as a result of brain damage brought on by the anemia.

So doctors abandoned folic acid as a cure and went back to using liver extract. Meanwhile, other scientists were working on liver to find the missing substance and they found it—vitamin B_{12} which, as we know today, is the substance in liver which cures and prevents pernicious anemia. Today Vitamin B_{12} is available for everyone to take. It is being used by many physicians as a treatment for general debility—"a shot of B_{12}" is accepted therapy in many physicians' offices for old folks or people with vague complaints of fatigue and ill health. Vitamin B_{12} is usually injected by doctors for, if you take it internally, you need very large amounts to equal the effects that one injection brings.

The reason for this brings us to the question of why some people get pernicious anemia to begin with. Dr. Murphy says that such people are born with a defect in the stomach wall which prevents the secretion of enough hydrochloric acid, a digestive juice. Without this, vitamin B_{12} is not absorbed from food. The reason it is absorbed from liver is because there is so much of the vitamin in liver, as compared to other food, that some of the vitamin gets through and is absorbed. But the treatment with B_{12} is always more effective if it is injected.

Dr. Murphy cautions his physician readers to test their patients for diminished amounts of hydrochloric acid in their stomachs, if they complain of numbness or tingling in hands and feet, weakness or becoming easily fatigued. For best results treatment must be continued throughout life, he says, and pernicious anemia patients, properly treated, often live longer than other people, because they take good care of themselves. It seems possible, too, that all the other nutritional goodies in liver, aside from the vitamin B_{12}, may contribute to this long life and good health. One patient of Dr. Murphy's still eats more than half a pound of broiled liver daily. She is 80 years old and in excellent health. Other patients who control their anemia with vitamin B_{12} also take liver frequently, he says, for they say it makes them feel better!

Dr. Murphy says he is convinced that there is something else in liver that takes part in the cure. "Liver and its extracts may contain something other than vitamin B_{12} that is necessary for control of all manifestations of the disease," he says. "Most of my patients treated with liver have not only had long lives but have been able to keep their jobs. Only those few in whom severe neural (nerve) problems developed before they started treatment have not been able to work."

We health-seekers have always known that food—real, whole, natural food—contains many healing factors that are not in individual vitamins and minerals. This is one reason why we recommend natural food supplements which contain at least a small part of the original food from which the supplement is made—the bioflavonoids that accompany the vitamin C in rose hips, the entire B complex of vitamins that is found in brewers yeast, wheat germ, desiccated liver.

As we grow older we tend to have less and less hydrochloric acid in our stomachs, which may result in pernicious anemia or other diseases involving lack of absorption of vitamins and minerals. This is one reason why older folks need more vitamin supplements than younger ones—they absorb less.

Finally, do we need any more evidence than Dr. Murphy provides in order to know that liver is one of our best foods—in fresh or desiccated form. Eat it at least once a week—oftener if you can. And for people who cannot or will not eat fresh liver, desiccated liver supplies the same nutritional goodies.

CHAPTER 3

No One Should Have Anemia

"THE FIFTH OF MAY is still celebrated as 'red crystal day' in my laboratory—the date in 1948 when the first microscopic crystals appeared of vitamin B_{12} isolated from liver. This newest vitamin still excites great interest among scientists." So says British scientist Dr. E. Lester Smith in an article in *New Scientist* for June 11, 1964. Dr. Smith, one of the world's foremost authorities on vitamin B_{12}, goes on to give us some facts on this most remarkable vitamin, which prevents pernicious anemia among other things.

It has the most complex chemical structure of any vitamin. It is the only vitamin to contain a metal (cobalt) and also phosphorus. Wherever it is found in nature, its source is microorganisms—that is, bacteria of one kind or another, for only these "lowly creatures" are able to manufacture this vitamin. It cannot be made synthetically in laboratories. Vitamin B_{12} is the most potent of known vitamins. Daily human requirements amount only to a few micrograms—and a microgram is one-millionth of a gram.

We do not know how vitamin B_{12} acts in our bodies. It is believed to be involved in the way we use protein, fats and carbohydrates. It performs some of its functions in connection with folic acid, but we know little as yet about this association. "Fortunately for those who need it," says Dr. Smith, "the vitamin does not have to be extracted from natural sources like liver . . . but is made by large scale fermentation procedures akin to those used for penicillin and other antibiotics . . . it is really one of the cheapest vitamins reckoned by dose."

As mentioned earlier, vitamin B_{12} and folic acid are important in preventing two kinds of anemia. Actually, the various types of anemia are ever present everyday problems among old folks, according to a British physician, Roger Lewis, writing in *Geriatrics*, December, 1976.

He quotes studies in England which show that 7.3 per cent of all elderly people have anemia. Other surveys turned up the information that, of 472 elderly people, 5.6 per cent of the men and 9.9 per cent of the women had anemia. Another survey done in 1973 brought to light the fact that 20 per cent of the women had anemia.

The incidence of anemia increases with advancing age. Among patients admitted to geriatric departments up to 40 per cent are anemic and the percentage of those with severe anemia more than doubles between the seventh and ninth decade of life. Those who are especially at risk are people who are over 75, housebound, living alone or mentally disturbed, or who have a history of anemia or surgery somewhere along the digestive tract.

Iron deficiency anemia is the most common kind. Iron is the trace mineral which keeps red blood cells healthy. This kind of anemia is caused mostly by loss of blood from some part of the digestive tract, possibly caused by hiatal hernia, peptic ulcers, diverticular disease, colon cancer or hemorrhoids.

Another common reason for iron deficiency anemia in older folks is the use of aspirin compounds and other pain killers and inflammation-fighters all of which can cause bleeding in the stomach or intestines. By this Dr. Lewis does not mean an occasional pill for a headache. Many arthritis patients are put on massive doses of aspirin by their doctors and this treatment goes on for life. All elderly people who have anemia should be questioned by the doctor, he says. If they are taking aspirin compounds regularly they should have regular tests for iron deficiency anemia.

Dr. Lewis also points out that older folks, in general, don't have as much to spend on food as younger folks. And foods in which iron is plentiful are expensive: meat, liver, eggs, leafy green vegetables and whole grains. Refined cereals, white bread and milk are relatively low in iron.

Among those who have had stomach surgery, 20 to 50 per cent of all patients become anemic within five years, probably because of frequent hemorrhages or inability to take enough food to get ample iron. The answer is to take iron supplements.

Another kind of anemia is pernicious anemia which appears in about one per cent of everybody over the age of 60. This has only one cause—lack of vitamin B_{12}. And, among older folks, says Dr. Lewis, the main reason for lack of vitamin B_{12} is lack of the digestive juice in the stomach (intrinsic factor) which is necessary to absorb this vitamin. But other conditions, as well, contribute to lack of B_{12}. Diverticulosis, abnormal formations of the colon and the wrong kind of bacteria in the colon. Several diseases (Crohn's disease for example) affect the lower part of the intestine where vitamin B_{12} is mostly absorbed.

Dr. Lewis believes it's easy to get enough B_{12} at meals, for only a very small amount of it is necessary—three micrograms per day is the standard requirement in our country. This vitamin is not destroyed by cooking or preserving and the liver stores considerable quantities of it. But it occurs only in foods of animal origin like liver, meat, milk and eggs, so vegetarians who eat no food of animal origin run a serious risk of getting pernicious anemia.

Lack of folic acid can cause a different kind of, but equally serious anemia. This is common among older people, says Lewis, and mostly because they just do not get enough of it in food. The best sources are leafy green vegetables and liver. It cannot be stored in the body longer than four months. Fifty to ninety per cent of it is lost in cooking. It is absorbed into the body from the upper part of the small intestine. This is the very part of that complicated mechanism where sensitivity to gluten occurs. Gluten is a protein in most cereal foods to which some people are allergic. Old folks who have this allergy do not generally suffer from the diarrhea which is the usual symptom, so they may not know that they are allergic to gluten. There are other ailments that make absorption of folic acid more difficult—leukemia, exfoliative dermatitis and treatment with drugs to control convulsive diseases like epilepsy.

Chronic kidney failure, chronic infections, cancer, rheumatoid arthritis, thyroid problems and chronic liver disease are other conditions that often accompany anemia in older folks. Another kind of very serious anemia has been treated with folic acid and another B vitamin, pyridoxine. It should always be remembered that the cause of anemia in elderly people is often mixed, says Dr. Lewis. These patients may have deficiencies in more than one nutrient essential to prevent anemia and they may have accompanying diseases that make absorption of these nutrients difficult or impossible.

Often older people never suspect that they have anemia and doctors do not interpret their symptoms as being symptoms of anemia. Circulatory, heart and mental problems are usually present. Swollen ankles, difficulty in getting your breath, giddiness, palpitations of the heart, and heart failure are all very common symptoms of anemia. If it is severe it can produce the agonizing pain of angina pectoris.

Anemia may appear to be senility because it causes symptoms which are characteristic of this mental condition: apathy, depression, confusion and general fatigue, all of which can lead to the self-neglect so often found among older folks. Often they complain of a sore tongue, lack of appetite, a "pins and needles" sensation in feet and legs, clumsiness, weakness and difficulty in walking. Inflammation of the tongue is quite common. There may be bone tenderness and black and blue marks.

Dr. Lewis gives patients as much as 200 milligrams of iron a day as treatment for iron deficiency anemia. He uses either ferrous sulfate or ferrous gluconate usually, for all iron preparations are more easily absorbed in the "ferrous" form. Side effects such as lack of appetite, vomiting, pain in the stomach, diarrhea and constipation can be managed, says he, by having the patient take the tablets with food or reducing the dose. "Slow-release" preparations are especially helpful, he believes.

And he thinks this kind of dosage should be continued for three months after the blood picture has returned to normal. If the condition that caused it (bleeding internally) cannot be cured, then it may be necessary to continue taking iron tablets indefinitely. If the patient cannot absorb iron by mouth, Dr. Lewis gives it by injection. He lists a number of unpleasant and dangerous side effects that may occur: headache, vomiting, fever, rapid heart beat, disorientation, dizziness, skin rashes, blood pressure that is too low, difficulty in breathing, inability to urinate, leukemia-like conditions and disturbances of lymph glands.

For vitamin B_{12} deficiency he gives injections of 1,000 micrograms twice a week for two weeks and possibly more frequent doses for several months, if the patient has troublesome nerve symptoms. Then 250 to 1,000 micrograms are injected every two months. He feels that giving vitamin B_{12} by mouth is useless in older people since they will probably not have the necessary stomach enzyme to absorb it. For folic acid deficiency he gives 5 milligrams three times daily and, if there is evidence that it is not being absorbed, he injects it.

The health seeker naturally prefers to prevent all these chronic anemic conditions that can lead to so much unpleasantness and ill health. What's the best way to do it? Diet is of the utmost importance. It is well to keep in mind that every mouthful of food you eat which does not contribute its proper share of nutrients is making the situation worse.

So the first thing to do is to cross off your grocery list all those foods which are just empty calories without a hint of iron, vitamin B_{12}, folic acid or any other essential nutrient. This means no more desserts except fresh fruits and occasional wholegrain confections, along with raisins, prunes and other dried fruits which are good sources of iron. It means no more white bread or processed cereals. Instead use only real wholegrain products, rich in iron, use seeds and seed foods like beans, lentils, soybeans—all good sources of iron. Meat and eggs are other good sources.

The leafy green vegetables are good sources not only of iron but also of folic acid as well as vitamins A and C so don't neglect them. The deeper green the color, the more nutrients they contain, so eat watercress, parsley, spinach, broccoli, chard and so on. Liver is the best source of both iron and vitamin B_{12}. Eat it at least once a week, oftener if possible. Yes, we know you have heard stories about the drugs and pesticides to which food animals are exposed. The liver is the detoxifier of the body and it tends to collect some of these undesirable things. But the wealth of nutriment in liver is unmatched in any other food and we feel certain that these nutrients compensate for the possible drawbacks.

Don't forget wheat germ and wheat bran. They are rich in iron and B vitamins and you should be eating them anyway because of their fiber content which will do a lot to normalize those colon bacteria which Dr. Lewis believes are so important in preventing anemia. Bran and wheat germ will help to correct any diarrhea or constipation that may result from iron medication.

And finally, look over the iron preparations at your health food store. There are lots of them, all well-planned, all harmless in suggested amounts. Vitamin B_{12} supplements are there, too, and most nutritionists believe that if you take *enough* B_{12} at least some of it will be absorbed, even in very elderly folks. Folic acid comes in many all-in-one vitamin preparations.

Don't allow unsuspected anemia to rob you of most of life's pleasure and make you into a dreary, confused, tired, disagreeable complainer. Prevent it before it has a chance to destroy you!

Gastroenterology reported in 1962 that laboratory rats on a diet deficient in iron soon lost their ability to absorb vitamin B_{12}. It is true, too, that people suffering from some chronic condition that does not permit them to absorb their food properly will almost inevitably be lacking in vitamin B_{12}. This means sufferers from diarrhea, dysentery, sprue, and people who have had part of their stomachs removed.

CHAPTER 4

Extra Vitamin B_{12} May Be Helpful During Pregnancy

A Massachusetts Institute of Technology study has demonstrated that pregnant animals which get more than average vitamin B_{12} have offspring which are larger, healthier and more resistant to disease than animals born to mothers who are getting only average amounts of this B vitamin.

Dr. Paul N. Newberne and Vernon R. Young reported in *Nature* for March 23, 1973 that they used two groups of pregnant laboratory rats and gave both of them the usual highly nourishing laboratory diet which contains everything these animals need to flourish. Then they gave half of the expectant mothers a bit more vitamin B_{12} than the other group received.

When the rat pups were born, those of the mothers who got the most vitamin B_{12} were larger. This advantage stayed with them during the entire first year of life. They also had more protein per body weight than did the pups whose mothers got only the average amount of B_{12}. The vitamin-enriched animals also showed more active liver enzymes. These are some of the substances which are brought into use when the body has toxic substances or germs to deal with and to render harmless. So, presumably, the second group of rats would be better able to resist infections and potential toxicity from chemicals, pollution and so on.

During the first years of life the animals which got the most B_{12} also had less mortality from every cause. The scientists believe that these very significant results can probably be applied to human beings. Apparently the human mother who gets less than enough vitamin B_{12} during pregnancy is likely to have children whose weight will be lower, whose general health will be worse and whose resistance to infection will be less effective than children of a mother who is getting enough and more than enough vitamin B_{12}.

Say the authors, "Questions about many of the unexplained illnesses in children and the wide variations among individuals in their resistance to disease may conceivably be answered by more intensive study of the prenatal nutrient needs of mother and her fetus."

Note, please, that the pregnant rats who were getting the average amount of vitamin B_{12} were not ill or decrepit or ailing in any way. They were apparently as healthy as all laboratory rats are—and that is probably considerably healthier than a similar group of human beings, since these animals are carefully watched, fed and watered, are protected from any kind of stress, pollution, noise or any other environmental circumstance which might affect the experiment.

But when additional vitamin B_{12} was added to their diets the entire performance of childbirth and the health of offspring was improved immeasurably. No other change was made in diet or environment. Just that tiny bit of added vitamin B_{12} made all the difference not only in weight and health of the offspring at birth, but right through their first years of life.

As one might expect, the authors of this paper go out of

their way to caution pregnant women not to "dose themselves" with large amounts of any vitamin. The B group of vitamins seem to work well together and should not be unbalanced by getting too much of only one, they say. We do not know why scientists who are supposedly doing such experiments for the eventual benefit of human beings, not rats, should feel it necessary to include such comments at the end of their report. Obviously the rats were not getting so much vitamin B_{12} that it harmed them in any way. Nor is there any record of any harm being done to human beings by vitamin B_{12} in considerably larger doses than the officially recommended dose. The B vitamins and vitamin C have been used in massive doses by many knowledgeable physicians for many purposes. They have brought nothing but benefit. They are water soluble, which means that any excess over what the body needs is harmlessly excreted.

Perhaps the MIT scientists have just uncovered another facet of what Dr. Roger J. Williams of the University of Texas called "supernutrition". In his fine book *Nutrition Against Disease* (published by Bantam Books), Dr. Williams tells us that no one has any idea of what the potential for health, longevity and well-being might be if all human beings were getting "supernutrition"—that is everything they need to be just reasonably healthy, plus more of all the good things—protein, vitamins and minerals. If there were ways to measure these things, he says, we might be able to design diets which would provide so much more of everything than we need just to get by that we could all live much longer, happier, healthier lives.

The experiment with vitamin B_{12} seems to show the truth of such a theory. Even good diets which apparently contain all that the animal or human being needs of every nutrient can be improved, apparently, to such an extent that far better health, growth and resistance to disease is achieved.

CHAPTER 5

Vitamin B_{12} and Sterility

A PHYSICIAN IN the Department of Pathology of the Royal Berkshire Hospital, Reading, England, conducted a significant investigation of the relationship of vitamin B_{12} to sterility and reported it in *The Lancet* for September 29, 1962.

Laboratory technicians assess a man's potential for fathering children by studying the condition of the sperm—the microscopic reproductive cell in the human semen which unites with the female reproductive cell to form the beginning of a new human being. In cases where the complaint is sterility (or inability to father children), the tiny sperm cells are generally found to be too few in number, unhealthful, or perhaps quite motionless, and, hence, lifeless.

It has been found that, when some of the millions of sperm cells are formed abnormally, there is also a decrease in the total number of sperm cells and in the number of cells that appear to be alive. So, says Dr. Alan A. Watson, it is believed that perhaps the sperm cells are not maturing normally. Cells, of course, mature, just as larger organisms do, and a cell which does not completely mature cannot function normally.

A veterinary doctor, writing in a breeder's journal, has

shown that the fertility of sperm being used for artificial insemination of cattle improved when vitamin B_{12} was added to it. Deciding that there might be some connection between vitamin B_{12} levels and sterility in human sperm, Dr. Watson tested 30 patients of a sterility clinic. He checked the vitamin B_{12} level in the sperm and compared it to that of the blood. The vitamin B_{12} level in the sperm of two persons who were known to be fertile was found to be higher than the blood levels. In cases where the sperm of the patient was found to be abnormal—that is, the cells were not normally formed—the vitamin B_{12} levels in the sperm were less than that of the blood.

Three of these had an absence of sperm or a serious lack of vitality in the remaining sperm. Dr. Watson believes that these tests show that vitamin B_{12} may be very intimately involved with the maturing of sperm cells. This seems to indicate that its presence or deficiency would be an important consideration in the treatment of sterility.

Commenting on Dr. Watson's findings in a later issue of *The Lancet* (October 13), Drs. A. A. Sharp and L. J. Witts of Oxford, England describe the case of a patient of theirs—a man of 35 whose marriage had been childless. The sperm cells of this patient showed no activity, so they would be unable to fertilize an egg cell. In addition, it was found that many of the cells were improperly formed.

When they did further tests on this patient, they found that his blood condition was very bad and he was suffering from pernicious anemia. Vitamin B_{12} is the usual treatment for pernicious anemia, so this patient was given injections of B_{12}. (Injections of this vitamin are often given because in some cases patients cannot absorb vitamin B_{12} if it is given by mouth.)

The level of vitamin B_{12} in his blood rapidly returned to normal. Six months later, examination of the sperm showed that 75 per cent were active and healthy. The sperm were also normally formed. Eighteen months after he had begun treatment, his wife had a healthy child.

It is well known to blood specialists, say these authors, that women who have developed pernicious anemia during the reproductive period quite often conceive when they are given vitamin B_{12} to treat the anemia, even though they have been childless before this. It is also well known, they say, that pernicious anemia may be present and unsuspected for some years before there are any symptoms of its presence.

So they suggest that, whenever the sperm cells appear to be defective, physicians should test the level of vitamin B_{12} in the blood to see if pernicious anemia is present.

Two American physicians, writing in the *American Journal of Medicine*, volume 243, page 27, 1962 report that they treated eight pernicious anemia patients with injections of vitamin B_{12} at six month intervals and found that they could control the anemia successfully this way! So it seems that

Vitamin B_{12} Content of Some Common Foods

(We give the number of micrograms in 100 grams, the average serving)

	Micrograms
Beef, kidney	18–55
Beef, liver	31-120
Beef, round	3.4–4.5
Bread, whole wheat	0.2–0.4
Cheese, American	0.6
Cheese, Swiss	0.9
Egg, 1 whole	0.3
Fish, haddock	0.6
Fish, sole	1.3
Ham	0.9–1.6
Milk, whole	0.3–0.5
Milk, powdered	1–2.6
Soybean meal	0.2

injections of this vitamin are powerful, indeed, and exert their beneficial effects for many months.

We are, of course, more interested in preventing a shortage of vitamin B_{12} which might lead to one of the conditions described above. Vitamin B_{12} occurs almost exclusively in foods of animal origin—meat, fish, eggs, milk products, poultry. It is especially abundant in liver—one reason for making certain you eat this fine food frequently.

How much vitamin B_{12} should you get every day? The latest official figure from the National Academy of Sciences is three micrograms daily for adults, less for infants and children. The AMA Council on Foods and Nutrition believes that 2 to 10 micrograms of the vitamin a day will suffice.

Here they are talking about "the average diet" of course, which means nothing to you if your individual diet is deficient in foods which contain vitamin B_{12}. There is also a problem of absorption with this vitamin and it is believed that deficiency in the vitamin is usually due to an inability to absorb it from the digestive tract rather than a lack in the diet.

If you are suffering from pernicious anemia your doctor will give you a substance called "the intrinsic factor" which appears to be essential for absorption of the vitamin. To prevent pernicious anemia and possibly sterility, see to it that you eat a good diet containing plenty of protein foods of animal origin. And eat liver at least once a week.

CHAPTER 6

Vitamin B_{12} Treats Skin Pigmentation

SKIN AND ALLERGY NEWS for November, 1973 tells of an eight-year old girl bothered with peculiar skin pigmentation. The mottled coloring appeared first on her fingers when she was only eight months old and gradually spread over the rest of her body. No doctors knew how or why her skin took on this coloring. No treatment brought relief. Then her doctor discovered that the child was suffering from pernicious anemia, the disease of deficiency in vitamin B_{12}. He gave her injections of the vitamin once a month and the pigmentation disappeared within 14 months.

Specialists still do not know how the vitamin is involved in skin pigmentation, but they say that apparently this child was born with a defect in her ability to use vitamin B_{12}. This apparently affected not just her blood, creating anemia, but also her entire body, including her skin. This story is a good example of what Dr. Roger Williams calls "biochemical individuality"—that is, the need for far greater amounts of some food element than others may need. In this case, the need was for far more vitamin B_{12} than the child's diet gave her.

It's interesting to note that many doctors tried unsuccessfully to treat the skin problem of this child, without ever uncovering the fact that she was deficient in vitamin B_{12}.

It seems quite likely the same thing may be true for many of us who have mysterious conditions which no doctor can diagnose or treat. Who knows? They may result from an undiscovered deficiency of a vitamin or mineral. The signs and symptoms of deficiency in most of the vitamins and minerals have been fairly well standardized. If doctors choose to look for them they will probably be able to discover these well-known standard signs and symptoms.

But what of obscure things like peculiar skin pigmentation? To our knowledge this has never been listed as a sign of deficiency in vitamin B_{12}. Yet it appears that this was the chief symptom of this child. Was she born with an inability to assimilate this B vitamin? Was she born with a need for far greater amounts of it than the rest of us? Was she, by chance, victim of a vegan diet (her own or her mother's) which deprived her of this B vitamin which is almost entirely lacking in purely vegetarian diets?

We do not know. But we do know that this vitamin is harmless even in very large amounts, as all the B vitamins are. We do know that all of us can and should be taking a supplement that contains it, as well as eating those foods in which it is most abundant. Who knows what other pesky, troublesome symptoms we may be able to overcome by just this one precaution?

CHAPTER 7

Vitamin B_{12} and Folic Acid Used to Treat Psoriasis

IT'S A SCALY DISEASE, the silvery scales affecting various parts of the body and in some cases, almost the entire body. There are 11 duly tabulated kinds and degrees of psoriasis: flexural psoriasis, psoriasis of the scalp, guttate psoriasis, erythrodermic psoriasis, pustular psoriasis of palms and soles of feet, generalized pustular psoriasis, psoriatic arthritis, psoriasis of the nails and mixed skin disorders, with psoriasis as one of the complications.

It is estimated that two to three per cent of us—four to eight million Americans—suffer from this disease, though we do not know for sure, since many victims of the disease conceal their condition because it is unsightly. More women than men suffer from psoriasis. Black Americans and West Africans are almost immune. Anything which disturbs the general health may initiate a flare-up of the skin condition. Anything which promotes a feeling of well-being and relaxation (a happy vacation, for example) tends to improve the condition.

Mostly it attacks people between the ages of 10 and 50.

Medical literature tells us solemnly that there is no cure and the disease will probably continue throughout life, although temporary remissions are to be expected.

Doctors give a number of drugs to psoriasis victims to take internally or apply to the affected areas. None of these is successful in every case and the most they can do is to control the disease, never cure it.

In the nutritional area, investigation has shown many helpful procedures. In 1964, *Medical World News* reported that two Russian physicians were getting excellent results with vitamin B_{12} combined with folic acid and vitamin C. The doctors treated 72 patients with injections of the above vitamins twice daily for 20 days. After a treatment-free period of three weeks, they gave the injections again for another 20 days. Good results followed the first course of treatment in 29 patients and after the second course of treatments in 25 patients and after the third course of treatment in four patients. The remaining 14 patients reported no improvement. Relapses occurred within six months in 52 patients and after six months in eight patients.

There seems to be no reason why these treatments could not have been prolonged since these vitamins are harmless. They could also have been taken by mouth.

A Brooklyn physician, writing to the *News* stated that he has been using B_{12} injcctions along with a proteolytic enzyme in resistant cases of psoriasis with "marvelous results". On the other hand a 1964 article in the *British Medical Journal* reported no success with vitamin B_{12} injections. This is the way nutritional treatment often turns out when it is given for short periods of time and when not enough of the vitamin is given. We do not know how much vitamin B_{12}, folic acid and vitamin C were given or for how long. Today we know that these water-soluble vitamins are harmless and can be taken in very large doses, with no risk. Perhaps this is essential in stubborn cases.

A London physician uses vitamin B_{12} to treat psoriasis. Dr. E. Lipman Cohen remarked on another physician's letter to the *British Medical Journal*, in which the former doctor said he had tried shots of B_{12} for psoriasis and they didn't work. Dr. Cohen said he gives his patients a total of 30 injections. He has never found a smaller number to be of any use. "Improvement is often delayed until up to six weeks after stopping treatment," he says. No doctor should give up on this therapy until they have used his dosage (1,000 micrograms) for 30 injections. Dr. Cohen's report appeared in the January 12, 1963 issue of the *British Medical Journal*.

A form of vitamin A applied to the skin controlled psoriasis, according to an article in the *Journal of the American Medical Association* for March 10, 1969. The University of Miami physicians used it on 26 patients with psoriasis, with excellent results. The doctors say they have read of psoriasis victims using vitamin A orally in doses which were toxic and not getting results. But when "vitamin A alcohol" was applied to the affected area in their tests, improvement was striking.

The *New York State Journal of Medicine* for November 1, 1973 reported the use of retinoic acid on psoriasis. This is a form of vitamin A for applying externally. It has also been used successfully for treating acne vulgaris. In 22 cases of psoriasis there was "significant improvement" after the skin treatment. Another article in the same journal described a case of severe liver damage caused by treating psoriasis with one of the drugs which doctors use.

There seems to be a close association between psoriasis, arthritis and diabetes as well as other disorders of blood sugar regulation. Along with an inherited tendency toward arthritis and diabetes, certain eating habits handed down from one generation to another seem to suggest that diets in which sugar plays too big a part may be involved in all these disorders. It's a simple thing to eliminate sugar in all forms from one's meals and see whether the psoriasis clears up. It's always wise to consider white sugar as a harmful drug and treat it as such. Just avoid it as you would a poison.

Several years ago some skin specialists got excited over the possibility that psoriasis might be caused by trouble with one of the amino acids, tryptophan. No one knows why, but apparently some psoriatics improve when this one amino acid is almost entirely removed from their diets. Mealtimes become somewhat monotonous, since the single high-protein food which contains no tryptophan is turkey. Most other foods contain it.

Two New York physicians, Dr. Harry Spiera and Dr. Albert M. Lefkovits, designed a low tryptophan diet which, they said, brought great improvement to a number of patients. One 19-year-old woman with psoriasis patches on face, chest, abdomen, arms and legs took the usual hospital diet for one week, then was placed on the low tryptophan diet. Her skin cleared in one week. Two weeks later she had no skin symptoms.

Another patient, a 46-year-old woman, had suffered from psoriasis for 17 years when she was put on the "turkey diet". Her psoriasis symptoms were relieved and scalp hair started to grow for the first time in 10 years. Whenever she goes off the "turkey diet" her psoriasis symptoms recur.

The point is not to add turkey to your usual diet. Turkey must become the main source of protein in your dict and it must be eaten every day at almost every meal. A typical day's diet outlined in *Medical World News* for October 13, 1967 recommends a breakfast of nothing but orange juice and coffee with heavy cream, lunch consists of grapefruit juice, steamed white meat of turkey, boiled potato, stewed tomatoes, pears, heavy cream, coffee and butter for cooking. Dinner is tomato juice, steamed white meat of turkey, boiled potato, butter, canned asparagus, grapefruit and coffee with heavy cream. In all cases the doctors gave niacin, the B vitamin, which is closely connected with the amino acid tryptophan and which must be taken if tryptophan is not in the diet, or the deficiency disease pellagra will result.

We have heard nothing about the turkey diet for several years, so we do not know whether it is still being prescribed. The diet outlined above is so low in protein and high in fat that it would seem quite dangerous to undertake it on one's own. It seems to us a far better idea might be to reconstruct one's diet along generally healthful lines and use as much white meat of turkey as possible in the diet, just to avoid the tryptophan in other poultry and meat. Turkey is one of the least expensive foods you can buy at present, so it should not be difficult to substitute it for meat and other poultry items.

Finally, we found a note indicating that levels of the trace mineral zinc are low in victims of psoriasis. *The Lancet* for November 11, 1967 reported on tests made of patients with psoriasis and those with leg ulcers and other skin diseases. The level of zinc in the blood of psoriatics and other skin patients was low. The British writers tell us that zinc deficiency in animals results in a condition like psoriasis.

Modern diets, high in refined sugar and starch invite zinc deficiency. Seventy-eight per cent of the zinc is removed from wholegrain flour when it is refined and none is returned to "enrich" flour. In the refining of sugar, 98 per cent of the zinc is removed and, of course, never returned. So people whose meals have included large amounts of desserts, doughnuts, cakes, candy, soft drinks, white bread, commercial cereals and pasta made from refined white flour are inviting zinc deficiency.

Says Dr. Henry Schroeder of Dartmouth Medical School in his book *Pollution, Profits and Progress,* "Pregnant women, women on The Pill, undernourished children, older people with disease of their arteries, and many others are deficient in zinc and the condition is relieved by taking zinc salts. Older people, people who drink alcohol regularly, and people on crackpot diets should probably take zinc salts, just as they take iron now. . . ." Zinc supplements are available today in health food stores.

And where do you get zinc, it you prefer to get it in food? Right where it was when they refined it out to make the commercial cereals and the white flour—in wholegrains. The official *Recommended Dietary Allowances* for 1974 have been revised to include zinc as an essential mineral. Adults need some 15 milligrams daily. Says the official booklet, "There are wide areas in the United States in which the soil is deficient in available zinc, and appearance of spontaneous zinc deficiency in farm animals has necessitated zinc enrichment of animal feeds." And farm animals, of course, are not fed on refined and processed starches. Unlike human beings, they are worth money, so they are fed high-quality protein grains which are always wholegrains. Even so, they may suffer from zinc deficiency when their food is grown in soil deficient in zinc.

Meat, liver, eggs, seafood (especially oysters) are excellent sources of zinc, as are milk and all wholegrain cereal and bread products. But it must be really wholegrain.

CHAPTER 8

Mental Illness and Vitamin B_{12}

YEARS AFTER vitamin B_{12} was discovered and found to be the magic potion that would prevent the hitherto untreatable and usually fatal disease of pernicious anemia, observant doctors and psychiatrists began to take closer notice of certain psychiatric symptoms that often appeared in people with pernicious anemia.

Little by little they discovered that these symptoms might appear in people who did not seem to have pernicious anemia, so had not been diagnosed as being deficient in vitamin B_{12}.

After tests were developed which would clearly demonstrate a deficiency in vitamin B_{12}, it was discovered, sure enough, that many people who were being diagnosed as mentally ill were suffering from nothing more serious than a deficiency in vitamin B_{12}, even though they did not have other symptoms of pernicious anemia.

Here are some of the notes about this strange circumstance that appeared in those early years and some that have appeared in later years. The lack of mention of vitamin B_{12} in most of today's professional material written for psychiatrists makes us wonder whether our psychiatrists have by now forgotten about the possibility that many of their psychiatric patients may be suffering from vitamin B_{12} deficiency and do not need expensive psychiatric care—just a "shot" of B_{12} once in a while.

In 1965 Irish physicians reported in *The Journal of the Irish Medical Association* on 12 cases in which the psychiatric picture "was associated" with low blood levels of vitamin B_{12}. The patients were perplexed and depressed. Doctors gave them every conceivable treatment for depression and got no results. They saw no symptoms of pernicious anemia so did not suspect it.

But tests of the patients' blood demonstrated low levels of vitamin B_{12}. The authors say that "further research may show a need for routine examinations of blood vitamin B_{12} levels in the older age group of psychiatric patients. Early diagnosis may prevent regression to an irreparable organic illness."

In 1965 *The Lancet* carried a letter from two London doctors on the mental symptoms in vitamin B_{12} deficiency.

They say, "Our experience of psychiatric practice suggests that nervous symptoms due to B_{12} deficiency occur about ten times more frequently than those due to syphilis. Therefore there seems to be better reason for performing in psychiatric patients routine screening tests for B_{12} deficiency than the Wassermann reaction and the Kahn tests."

They have seen an increasing number of patients with vitamin B_{12} deficiency, they say, including 14 patients with a history of partial removal of the stomach who were admitted to a mental hospital because of psychiatric symptoms. Two of them were found to be lacking in vitamin B_{12}. The doctors feel strongly, they say, that anyone who has a history of dyspepsia (indigestion) or surgery should be tested for vitamin B_{12} deficiency, even if they are not anemic.

A 1965 editorial in *The Lancet* summarized the information available up to then regarding mental and psychiatric symptoms in vitamin B_{12} deficiency.

"Frank psychoses have been reported in between four per cent and 16 per cent of patients," the editorial says, "taking all forms from confusional states to affective conditions, although several workers note a tendency to paranoid symptoms." That is, a feeling of being persecuted.

One researcher reported that over a third of nearly 1,500 patients examined had psychiatric symptoms "manifest to even a casual observer." Such changes were irritability, mental apathy, fluctuations of mood. Other characteristics are abnormal readings in electroencephalograms, (up to two-thirds of the cases) alterations in brain metabolism, and pathological changes in the brain.

It was pointed out, too, that psychiatric symptoms can precede any other signs of vitamin B_{12} deficiency. In one study, four out of 25 patients had psychological symptoms for up to eight years before the doctors diagnosed pernicious anemia. Another doctor recorded a further six cases which he called "megaloblastic madness". Megaloblastic refers to the kind of blood cells found in individuals with pernicious anemia.

Mental illness due to vitamin B_{12} deficiency is not common, says the author of the editorial, but it is readily treated and, as in other kinds of mental illness, it may take many forms. So tests for levels of vitamin B_{12} in the body are essential. Today, fortunately, we have such tests.

In a 1966 issue of *The Lancet* a physician at a mental hospital in Copenhagen reported on tests made of all patients admitted above the age of 65. With one exception, all levels of vitamin B_{12} in the blood *were below normal in all elderly patients*. Examination of a group of younger patients showed higher levels of vitamin B_{12}.

A 1961 issue of *The British Medical Journal* speaks of the symptoms of B_{12} deficiency—symptoms which vary in severity from mild disorders of mood, mental slowness and memory defects to severe psychotic symptoms, including agitation, depression, severe confusional and hallucinatory states and paranoid behavior. Such symptoms may precede by several years any indication of anemia or other conditions resulting from vitamin B_{12} deficiency.

In 1969 a West German medical journal once again reminded physicians the world over that emotional disturbances, psychoses and neurological (nerve) signs are frequent occurrences in vitamin B_{12} deficiency. The psychoses are usually reversible, said these three physicians, and may range from mild transitory disorders to loss of consciousness. They urged their psychiatric colleagues to give tests for vitamin B_{12} to all patients entering mental hospitals.

The July 1, 1967 *British Medical Journal* reported on a 53-year-old woman brought to the hospital because of numbness and tingling in arms and legs which had been diagnosed as being due to rheumatic troubles in her neck. She was put into traction with "partial relief."

Four days after she was admitted to the hospital she suddenly became psychotic, totally confused, with paranoid delusions and hallucinations that she was hearing things that were not there. She believed that others in the ward were saying derogatory things about her and that she was about to undergo a serious brain operation. None of which was true.

The doctors injected vitamin B_{12} and, within 24 hours, she began to improve, was completely over her psychotic imaginings in 48 hours.

In *Nutrition Against Disease,* Dr. Roger J. Williams has this to say: "Vitamin B_{12} is definitely a link in the nutritional chain that protects against mental disease. In pernicious anemia, the mental symptoms are by no means uniform; they can range from such mild symptoms as having difficulty in concentrating or remembering to stuporous depression, severe agitation, hallucinations, or even manic or paranoid behavior.

"Like the symptoms in pellagra," continued Dr. Williams, "those caused by B_{12} deficiency may be very similar to those observed in schizophrenia. Yet the relationship between pernicious anemia and B_{12} is not simple; other factors may be involved as well. Sometimes administering B_{12} will clear up the mental symptoms associated with pernicious anemia rather slowly—and, occasionally, incompletely. The relationship between vitamin and disease is not as direct as in the case of pellagra."

The 69-year-old-woman was brought to a hospital with a history of pallor, fatigue, forgetfulness and lack of energy. On the day before, she fell in her apartment and could not get up because of weakness. Hospital attendants found it difficult to awaken her. She said she ate meat daily and fresh fruit and vegetables at least three times a week. The hospital physicians gave her a complete battery of tests in an effort to diagnose her condition. There seemed to be no doubt that she was suffering from megaloblastic anemia, with diseased blood cells and other symptoms characteristic of the anemia caused by lack of vitamin B_{12}.

But the patient had been given an injection of vitamin B_{12} the week before she came to the hospital, and her blood levels of this essential vitamin were high. So something else was obviously wrong. The doctors gave her folic acid, the B vitamin closely related to B_{12}. She began to improve at once and was soon discharged from the hospital. Tests taken six months later showed her in good health. Her mind was clear. She walked normally. Her fatigue and forgetfulness were gone.

The authors of this article, in the *Journal of the American Medical Association* for July 31, 1972 point out that there was a history of pernicious anemia in her family. They tell us of two other elderly patients whose "dementia" was cured by giving them folic acid.

One would think that tales of such cases would disappear from medical journals now that all physicians must be aware of the possibility of such things happening. But we read in *Archives of Internal Medicine* for October, 1971 of a Washington, D. C. woman who was brought to the hospital with psychotic symptoms which the doctors did not suspect could be caused by lack of a vitamin until they tested her for vitamin B_{12}. Sure enough, that was all that was the matter with her. She was well in eight days after vitamin B_{12} therapy.

Says the physician, "It may be desirable to measure serum vitamin B_{12} routinely in all new mentally disturbed patients."

We doubt that it is being done. A visit at any nursing home reveals many many guests suffering from just the symptoms described above. Wandering aimlessly through the halls, these elderly people are confused about almost everything. Many are convinced that those around them are bent on harming them or stealing from them. Many have hallucinations and other more serious indications of mental problems. Mostly they seem to be given tranquilizers which, after a time, appear to make their symptoms worse.

If you have a family member who is developing any of the mental symptoms described above, by all means try to discover if he or she is suffering from a deficiency in vitamin B_{12}. Even if there is no evidence of this ask the doctor to try a series of vitamin B_{12} injections, which are totally harmless and, perhaps, may be all that is necessary to bring the individual back to good mental health. Injections are usually recommended because elderly folks have more difficulty than the rest of us in absorbing vitamin B_{12} from their meals. And peculiar dietary habits developed over many years may have made their diets very low in vitamin B_{12}.

CHAPTER 9

Lack of Vitamin B_{12} Is a Threat to Some Vegetarians

IN RECENT YEARS many health-conscious folks, as well as those with strict ethical principles against using animal products, have enthusiastically embraced vegetarianism as a way of life.

Many such newly convinced vegetarians have maintained themselves and their families in good health, so long as they observed the rules of combining vegetarian foods to best advantage where complete protein is concerned. Since all vegetarian foods are short in one or more amino acids or links of protein, combining complementary foods at the same meal results in what dieticians call "complete protein," meaning that all the essential amino acids are present in sufficient quantity to bring such a vegetarian meal up to the level of protein in foods of animal origin like meat, fish, poultry, eggs and dairy products.

So long as any food of animal origin is eaten at a vegetarian meal, there is little chance of "wasting" protein by not providing enough complementary food to make complete protein. Eggs, milk, cheese or yogurt in any form added to dishes prepared for a vegetarian meal, or eaten along with the vegetarian meal guarantee sufficient complete protein for good health.

Those vegetarians called "vegans", however, do not eat any food that comes from an animal source. This leaves them open to deficiencies in those food elements that are present only in foods of animal origin. The two of these with which we are most familiar are vitamin B_{12} and vitamin D. Adults on totally vegan diets, it appears, can manage to get along on very small amounts of these vitamins. But it's different with children.

In 1976 British medical journals reported on an epidemic of pernicious anemia (caused by lack of vitamin B_{12}) in vegetarian people who had emigrated from Asia to England and were still eating their traditional diet in England.

Dr. Michael Rose of St George's Hospital Medical School in London reported in the September 25, 1976 issue of *The Lancet* that deficiency in vitamin B_{12} is now a recognized cause of a serious kind of anemia (megaloblastic) among the Hindu community of recent immigrants to England. It is "commonplace", he says, in some communities where Asians live. One doctor identified more than 500 cases among the Asian patients at one hospital between 1970 and 1975. In most cases the anemia problems disappear with oral vitamin B_{12}, so it seems probable that there is no problem with absorbing the vitamin. These folks are just not getting any in their food.

Dr. Rose believes that the packaging and methods of hygiene used in preparing commercial food for stores in England may have something to do with this widespread epidemic. Obviously these Hindu people did not suffer from vitamin B_{12} deficiency in their homeland or, over the centuries, they would have developed some adaptation of diet or food preparation which would have prevented the anemia.

"One can only assume," says Dr. Rose, "that the methods

of hygiene and packaging adopted in this country wash off all the residual vitamin B_{12} contaminating the vegetable produce."

This suggests that food raised without pesticides and not washed may contain enough in the way of tiny insects (aphids, for example) to provide vitamin B_{12} for those who eat it. Food grown in Britain, with pesticides, then washed probably in several waters with, perhaps, detergent included before marketing would destroy all such sources of vitamin B_{12}.

Dr. Rose says that the best solution is to talk to the mother of the family or whatever relative prepares the food explaining the problem and asking her to sprinkle over a family meal once a month a single capsule of vitamin B_{12}—one milligram. He believes this is enough vitamin B_{12} to assure the health of the entire family, for we need very little of this vitamin for good health.

He tells the story of one woman who came to him with pernicious anemia. Her husband had been treated for the same trouble six months earlier. But no one, apparently, had explained to this woman what had caused her husband's trouble or how easy it is to avoid such health disasters.

Dr. Rose's article sparked a number of letters from other readers of *The Lancet*. In the October 30, 1976 issue a member of the Vegetarian Society pointed out that it is not necessary for dedicated vegetarians to use milk or eggs to get their vitamin B_{12}. A yeast extract sold in England contains it, he said, and some vegetarian foods made of vegetable textured protein "offer acceptable and convenient low-fat sources of the vitamin, suitable for inclusion in traditional dishes such as curries."

Dr. M. Swash of London wrote in to describe the case of a Ugandan Asian who had been in England for only two months when he noticed burning sensations in both legs and an unsteady gait. During the next six months he lost the ability to walk at all. The doctor discovered that levels of vitamin B_{12} in his blood were very low. He was given injections of vitamin B_{12} and tablets to take orally.

He also agreed to include some dairy products and eggs in his meals. He improved rapidly. The London doctor points out that there were only slight indications of blood disorder in this patient—the disorders that one would expect with pernicious anemia. But the nerve symptoms were "severe".

Dr. Swash believes that a long-standing marginal vitamin B_{12} balance became disturbed when this man moved to England from Africa. He says that monkeys kept in captivity also develop vitamin B_{12} deficiency, although they are healthy living in the open. "It has been suggested," says the doctor, "that vegans living in India obtain vitamin B_{12} from legumes or even from polluted well water and . . . such sources of vitamin B_{12} are probably not available in Britain." East Indians in their native country do not suffer from this deficiency.

Nevertheless, says Dr. Swash, whenever a patient comes in with a paraplegia—an inability to walk normally—vitamin B_{12} state should be investigated even though his or her blood may not show any indications of pernicious anemia.

In a later *Lancet*, two West German doctors describe a patient with a five-months history of slowly increasing paralysis of both legs. More than six years earlier he became mentally ill, broke off all contacts with family and friends, gave up his work and went on a diet without any food of animal origin, eating only fruit, vegetables, nuts and coffee.

He did not speak to the doctor when he was brought in for treatment and avoided looking at him. He appeared to be indifferent to the severity of his condition. He was suffering from both blood and nerve complications. Because there appeared to be no sign of lack of absorption from his digestive tract, he was given vitamin B_{12} by mouth. His pernicious anemia disappeared rapidly and his paralysis gradually improved. His frame of mind did not change, however. He remained anti-social, refused to give up his inadequate diet and refused to concede that diet had anything to do with his condition.

A final letter in this series came from a British doctor who pointed out the great difficulty doctors have in persuading complete vegetarians to include just a couple of glasses of milk in their diets. This would be enough, he says, to prevent the anemia.

When lack of vitamin B_{12} in food is combined with an inability to absorb whatever vitamin B_{12} is present, results can be disastrous, as witness a case described in *Nutrition Reviews* for August, 1978.

A 57-year-old man came to a hospital complaining of difficulty in walking for about three months prior to admission. Four years previously he had partially retired because he became tired so easily. He had not used any meat, fish, coffee or alcohol for the previous 25 years and had also avoided eggs and most dairy products during this time. He could justly be called a vegan. He took no vitamin supplements.

His family history was rather ominous. His mother was diabetic. His brother and sister, who followed a similar diet, but a bit less restricted, took vitamin supplements and had no health problems.

Two years before he came to the hospital the man had lost weight, suffered from lack of balance, dizziness and swollen ankles. Unfortunately he was advised to go on a fast, drink carrot juice and not take any vitamin B_{12}. He was told to eliminate dairy products entirely and use one raw egg yolk every other day.

He began to eat carrots and drink large amounts of carrot juice every day. A year later he developed a peculiar way of walking, numbness in hands and feet, loss of positional sense and impairment of the sense of touch. Very concerned, he began to take vitamin B_{12}—100 micrograms a day, along with the B vitamin niacin, iron and vitamin E. He did not improve.

The doctors at the hospital found his skin colored bright yellow from the carrot juice. He stopped taking it and the color disappeared. The doctors found that his hands and his legs below the knees were suffering from inability to feel sensations, even pinpricks. His feet were swollen. His blood levels of vitamin B_{12} were 146 units, compared to the normal level of 150 to 199. Not bad for someone who had been getting almost no vitamin B_{12} for most of his life. But the impairment in arms, hands and legs persisted.

The doctors gave him injections of 1,000 micrograms of vitamin B_{12} every day for three weeks. His blood and nerve conditions returned to normal rapidly. Monthly injections of vitamin B_{12} were continued for six months. He was then given 100 micrograms of B_{12} orally every day. By this time all symptoms had cleared, except for some lack of feeling in his feet.

He altered his diet to include tuna, milk, cheese, cereal and eggs. The level of vitamin B_{12} in his blood increased to 300 units—considerably above normal.

The doctors were interested in finding out just how much vitamin B_{12} was in the diet this man had been eating for so many years. So he went to the store and bought all the food he might eat in a day. The laboratory tested the whole batch of food for vitamin B_{12}.

Here are the foods he ate in a single day. Three bananas, two apples, one pear, servings of celery, lettuce, cabbage, kohlrabi, tomato, beet, turnip, green pepper, cucumber, plus nuts, one can of Campbell's vegetarian soup and one container of imitation vanilla ice cream, one processed American cheese sandwich on rye toast and one peanut butter and jelly sandwich on rye toast.

The laboratory found that the day's total of vitamin B_{12}

in all this food was 1.2 micrograms of vitamin B_{12}. A microgram is one-millionth of a gram. Says *Nutrition Reviews*, "This presumably represented the maximum vitamin B_{12} intake because on many days dairy products, which probably provided most of the vitamin B_{12} were not eaten."

The official Recommended Dietary Allowance for vitamin B_{12} is 3 micrograms. The patient was getting less than one-half of that and on many days not even that much, probably.

He was asked to cooperate in an examination of his ability to absorb vitamin B_{12}. He entered the hospital and the tests began. Seven months after intensive vitamin B_{12} therapy, the test which indicated his ability to absorb the vitamin from his digestive tract was abnormal. The substance called "intrinsic factor" which is essential for absorption of this vitamin was measured at 65 units per hour, compared with normal values of more than 1,000 units per hour.

Say the authors of this article, had the patient been able to absorb the very small amount of vitamin B_{12} his vegan diet provided, it's possible that he might have been able to avoid health problems. This is what occurs in most vegans, the authors believe, so they are able to maintain themselves healthfully on diets in which there is almost no vitamin B_{12}.

But in this patient the lack of digestive substances in his stomach which are essential for absorbing this vitamin and the lack of normal hydrochloric acid levels in his stomach produced the painful and disabling symptoms for which he had to seek help. And even four months after he was getting enough vitamin B_{12} by mouth and by injection, the digestive conditions did not improve. He was still unable to absorb more than a very small amount of this vitamin.

Most likely, say the authors, very low levels of vitamin B_{12} in meals bring on a precarious vitamin B_{12} balance, but somehow not quite enough to produce symptoms of ill health. But when digestive juices dry up and the specific compound that helps in the absorption of vitamin B_{12} is absent, then a serious deficiency state develops.

We are not told why this man decided to undertake such a strict vegetarian diet. We do not know if he might have been better off had he been balancing amino acids at every meal—that is, combining foods so that all the essential amino acids or links of protein would have been present at any given meal, so that he would have the optimal amount of complete protein at that meal.

Eating nuts or seeds with cereals or breads is one way to do this. Eating legumes (beans, peas, lentils, soybeans) at the same meal with cereals and breads, or with nuts and seeds at the same meal is another way to do this. Eating some food of animal origin at every meal is still another way—that is, eat some milk or cheese, one or two eggs at the same time you are eating an all vegetarian meal.

A baby fed nothing but breast milk from his vegan mother can develop symptoms of pernicious anemia, which is the disease resulting from lack of vitamin B_{12}. The nursing mother may show no symptoms of B_{12} deficiency. So she has apparently enough of this nutrient for her own needs, but not enough to provide for the baby's needs in her milk.

Now we have evidence, from responsible sources, that lack of vitamin D can also be a problem with children of vegans. Vitamin D is a fat soluble vitamin which some researchers think should be called a hormone rather than a vitamin, since the body manufactures vitamin D when bare skin is exposed to sunlight. A substance akin to cholesterol in the skin creates the vitamin from the ultraviolet light of the sun.

However babies kept indoors or wrapped in so much clothing that their skin is not exposed to sunlight do not have this source of vitamin D. The vitamin is essential for controlling the body's use of calcium and phosphorus, necessary minerals for bone growth and sturdy teeth.

The American Journal of Diseases of Children, in its February 1979 issue, reported on studies by a New England physician and an Israeli physician who studied the children of vegans—not the vegans themselves.

Dr. Johanna Dwyer of Boston's New England Medical Center and a group of colleagues studied 84 vegetarian children from vegan families of practicing yogas and Seventh-Day Adventist groups. They found two well-defined cases of rickets and indications of approaching rickets in 17 other children on strict vegetarian diets. They also reported two other cases of rickets in vegetarian children not in the original group.

Rickets is a disease which deforms. It is not hard to diagnose. It is so uncommon in today's babies that pediatricians seldom see a case or report a case to the medical journals. The long bones, chiefly those of the legs, are bowed, irretrievably. Pelvic bones in young girls may be so deformed that successful pregnancy will be impossible in later life. Wrists, ankles, and other parts of the skeleton may be deformed. The child may not attain full growth.

In Israel Dr. Fhud Zmora of Ben-Gurion University reported on four cases of rickets in the "Black Hebrew" community, a group of strict vegetarians who refuse any medical assistance except to save a life.

The four children examined had severe rickets and brittle bones. One of the children later died. The other improved somewhat after they were given vitamin D along with the minerals necessary to strengthen bones.

We do not know how these children were dressed or how often they were taken outside. It seems likely that the abundant sunshine of a country like Israel should have provided them with ultraviolet light for manufacturing enough vitamin D for good health. Perhaps their parents did not understand the necessity of exposure to sunlight. Reports from England have told of many cases of rickets in vegetarian children from East Indian parents born in England where the climate is cloudy and rainy. In winter not enough sunlight is available to supply vitamin D and the mothers of these children do not understand the necessity of taking a vitamin D supplement.

Most dairy milk in our country is irradiated with ultraviolet light to produce about 400 units of vitamin D per quart. Vitamin D is also added to many other foods in order to make certain that our babies and children get enough of it. But in a vegan family these foods are not eaten, so there is a good chance that babies may suffer lifelong deformities from lack of this vitamin.

The official recommendation of vitamin D for babies is 400 units a day—or what is contained in one quart of milk. In addition, pediatricians always counsel mothers to take their children out into the open air every sunny day. It is not necessary to "sunbathe"—in fact it is inadvisable to bake oneself brown with sunburn. There is plenty of ultraviolet light available on a sunny day beneath trees or in light shade. But the baby should not be bundled up so long as it is warm. The ultraviolet light must fall on bare skin in order to guarantee the manufacture of vitamin D.

Vitamin D from fish liver oil is inexpensively available at the health food store. Surely any vegan mother should be encouraged to give her baby this excellent source of vitamin D, especially in winter in northern parts of the country where

COMBINE

grains, cereals, pasta, bran, wheat germ, bread, muffins, biscuits, etc.	*with*	legumes such as soybeans, peas, beans, lentils, peanuts	*with*	nuts and seeds such as almonds, walnuts, sunflower seeds, etc.

almost no sunlight is available for many months.

In preparing vegan meals, the rules for combining different kinds of high protein foods are listed in the table, according to the balance of amino acids in each group. (Page 55.)

Combine any food from one column in the table with any food from other columns at the same meal, either in the same dish or a supplementary dish.

For those vegetarians who use dairy products and eggs, meal planning is greatly simplified since milk, yogurt, any kind of cheese and eggs prepared in any way contribute complete protein to the meal. However, in order to economize on precious protein and waste not a gram of it, the foods must be eaten at the same meal. Toast for breakfast and eggs for lunch is wasteful of protein. The protein of the toast has no other high protein food to complement it, so it is not used by the body. A glass of milk, a piece of cheese or an egg at breakfast render the protein of the toast available as complete protein to the body.

The best books we have ever found for explaining just how and why all this works in planning vegetarian diets are: *Diet for a Small Planet* by Frances Moore Lappé, and *Recipes for a Small Planet* by Ellen Buchman Ewald, both paperbacks published by Ballantine Books in New York City. Your health food store undoubtedly has these books on its shelves.

CHAPTER 10

Vitamin B_{12} and Vitamin C Are Not Antagonists

SEVERAL YEARS AGO a nutrition scientist, Dr. Victor Herbert, published a paper in the *Journal of the American Medical Association* announcing that anyone taking vitamin C at mealtime was likely to be short on vitamin B_{12} since vitamin C has a destructive action on the B vitamin. The implication is that the more vitamin C you take the less vitamin B_{12} you are going to have in your blood.

Vitamin B_{12} is essential to good health. It is present in any appreciable amount only in foods of animal origin, like meat, eggs, milk and, mostly, liver. People who don't eat much of such foods risk a vitamin B_{12}-shortage in any case. This can eventually lead to pernicious anemia, a disease so serious that it was usually fatal before doctors found out that it was caused by a simple lack of a vitamin.

So, understandably, some people who take lots of vitamin C were upset by the information on vitamin B_{12} and vitamin C which appeared in newspapers across the country. It seemed obvious to us that the many people who have been taking massive doses of vitamin C for many years are not perishing from pernicious anemia. And those of us who came later to a recognition of the value of large amounts of vitamin C are not experiencing symptoms of vitamin B_{12} deficiency.

Now we have a report from Fordham Hospital and Hoffman-LaRoche in which a carefully controlled laboratory test was done to test the stability of vitamin B_{12} in the presence of large amounts of vitamin C. The four researchers reported on their experiment in *The American Journal of Clinical Nutrition* for June, 1976.

They describe in detail the methods they used, so that any other scientist can use these same methods and check their results. They tested the vitamin B_{12} content of a meal with relatively high content of vitamin B_{12} and a meal with not nearly so much of the B vitamin. They added vitamin C up to half a gram (500 milligrams). They tell us that they could detect no destruction of vitamin B_{12} by the vitamin C.

The doctors point out that vitamin B_{12} is very stable in foods since it is bound closely to a protein in the food—so closely that "a prolonged chemical attack" could be withstood and the vitamin B_{12} would not be separated out and destroyed. So vitamin C simply cannot get to the B vitamin and destroy it.

They believe that the results gotten by the earlier scientists who reported destruction of vitamin B_{12} were brought about by the use of inadequate methods of extracting the B vitamin from the food being tested. By using, in the present experiment, standardized and official methods, they discovered that no appreciable vitamin B_{12} had been destroyed by the vitamin C.

We think you can feel perfectly confident that this test was done in good faith. It can easily be repeated to confirm it. If you are still doubtful about the possibility of losing some vitamin B_{12}, why not pop a vitamin B_{12} tablet into your mouth every few days? Or buy an all-in-one supplement which contains vitamin B_{12}. The amount in food is so very little that almost any level of vitamin B_{12} in a supplement is enormous by comparison. And there is no chance of an overdose. Vitamin B_{12}, like all B vitamins, and vitamin C, is water-soluble.

After Dr. Herbert published his claim, Dr. Jean Mayer, the syndicated columnist who is now president of Tufts University, published a column repeating Dr. Herbert's claim that vitamin C destroys vitamin B_{12}. We wrote to Dr. Mayer asking how this could be, since both are contained in liver. He did not answer.

In the April 21, 1975 issue of *The Journal of the American Medical Association,* five physicians from the Veterans Administration Hospital of the St. Louis University Group Hospitals wrote describing the condition of paraplegics in their spinal cord injury service. Paraplegics have special problems with urinary infections. Urinary infections can be troublesome and, in some cases, fatal. If they are not prevented in some way, it may be necessary to take various antibiotics for long periods of time, which can have side effects on other aspects of health.

So, say the St. Louis specialists, "As a routine procedure, all of the spinal cord injury patients on our service receive doses of (vitamin C) of more than 4 grams a day (4,000 milligrams) to enhance urinary acidity." The healthy urine is acid in character, rather than alkaline. This acidity helps to control bacteria.

In the St. Louis hospital, 10 patients aged 17 to 69 had been getting 4,000 milligrams of vitamin C daily for 11 months. All of them were on unrestricted diets and they got the vitamin in four doses during the day. This is considered the best way to take large doses of vitamin C, for the body excretes whatever excess is not needed about every four hours. So, to keep cells suffused with vitamin C constantly, it is best to take the vitamin every four hours or so—say, with every meal and again at bedtime.

When the St. Louis doctors read Dr. Herbert's warnings about vitamin B_{12}, they gave their paraplegic patients tests for vitamin B_{12}. They found in all cases that the levels of this B vitamin were high in their blood and in three cases were very high.

Dr. Herbert was asked by the *JAMA* to reply to this letter. He said in reply that it's possible the St. Louis assay for vitamin B_{12} could be in error and giving results that are too high. Are you sure, he asked, that these patients don't have something also the matter with them which might cause the levels of vitamin B_{12} to go up in their blood although other parts of their bodies were not getting enough of it to prevent anemia? This seems to us like childish quibbling. Obviously patients under the constant daily supervision of skilled experts are not going to pine away from pernicious anemia without somebody noticing it.

Furthermore, Dr. Herbert said that he never said that everybody getting lots of vitamin C is going to develop pernicious anemia from the lack of B_{12}. "It is quite possible that a group of patients could be taking 4 grams of ascorbic acid daily without developing vitamin B_{12} deficiency . . . moderate amounts of iron in the diet reduce the damaging effect of ascorbic acid on vitamin B_{12} and taking ascorbic acid between meals would be less damaging than taking it with meals." And, of course, he goes on, if anybody is taking vitamin B_{12} supplements then he would most likely *not* suffer from a deficiency in this vitamin if he's also taking vitamin C.

So much for the sensational headlines. Too bad everybody who read them can't also read what almost boils down to a retraction on the part of Dr. Herbert. If any of our readers are still worried about becoming anemic from taking too much vitamin C, just be sure you eat liver frequently (it has lots of vitamin B_{12}) or take desiccated liver or take a vitamin B_{12} supplement.

CHAPTER 11

Cobalt—The Most Important Part of Vitamin B_{12}

COBALT IS A silver-white metallic trace mineral occurring in compounds, the silicates, which give us important blue pigments for coloring things like pottery. The term Cobalt Blue is used for these pigments.

Until quite recently in modern nutritional history no one had any idea that cobalt might be important for human health or if it might even be toxic. In 1929 two researchers reported that cobalt in large doses affects blood cells in rats and induces a great increase in the number of red blood cells.

Scientists and veterinarians were interested, the latter because they were puzzled by a mysterious disease of sheep called "coast disease" or "wasting disease". By 1935 they had discovered that this disease, which was costly to sheepgrowers, was caused by lack of cobalt in the animals' diet. And the deficiency came about because of lack of the mineral in the soil on which their food was grown.

Says Dr. E. J. Underwood in *Trace Elements in Human and Animal Nutrition,* "The appearance of a severely cobalt deficient animal is one of extreme emaciation and listlessness, indistinguishable from that of a starved animal, except that the visible mucous membranes are blanched and the skin is pale and fragile. The emaciation or wasting of the musculature . . . results from the failure of appetite which is an early and conspicuous feature of the disease, and the paleness of the skin and mucous membranes from the anemia which usually develops progressively with the severity of the deficiency."

In one of the most crazy, mixed-up detective stories of all nutrition science, it was discovered in 1948 that the nutritional factor which could cure pernicious anemia in human beings was a compound containing the trace mineral cobalt.

So how is the soil deficiency in cobalt related to pernicious anemia and vitamin B_{12}? Another detective story. Scientists thought that vitamin B_{12} might be the functional form of cobalt in animals which eat and digest their food as sheep and cattle do—the ruminant animals, that is. The next time cobalt deficiency caused the "wasting disease" in lambs, they injected the lambs with vitamin B_{12} and cured the affliction. Apparently the animals were unable to synthesize enough vitamin B_{12} to keep themselves healthy when they weren't getting enough cobalt in their food!

There is no evidence of cobalt deficiency in human beings, even in parts of the world where there is not enough cobalt in the soil to keep ruminant animals healthy. "The significance of cobalt in human health and nutrition is confined, so far as it now is known, to its presence in vitamin B_{12}," says Dr. E. J. Underwood. "All ordinary diets supply much more cobalt than can be accounted for as vitamin B_{12} and no relationship necessarily exists between their cobalt and their vitamin B_{12} contents."

Green leafy vegetables contain more cobalt than other foods, with dairy products and refined cereals the poorest sources. Vitamin B_{12} is found chiefly in products of animal source: liver, meat, eggs.

Dr. Underwood tells us that the value of cobalt therapy in high blood pressure has been investigated. Cobalt salts produce "flushing" in human beings, which indicates that blood vessels have been dilated. This is the same reaction one gets from large doses of the B vitamin niacin. Two scientists treated nine high blood pressure patients with 50 milligrams of cobalt chloride a day for 10 to 65 days.

Three of the patients had a lowering of blood pressure to normal. Five had a 14 to 72 per cent reduction in the requirement for drugs to control their blood pressure. There were no toxic effects noted in any of these people.

We have not been able to find any follow-up experiments along these lines and we cannot give any guarantee that taking large amounts of vitamin B_{12} (containing cobalt) will do anything about lowering one's blood pressure. Fifty milligrams of cobalt is probably a lot more cobalt than you would get in even massive doses of B_{12}. If it's the cobalt in B_{12} that brings down blood pressure, however, it seems possible that taking B_{12} in every day's supplements might have a beneficial effect on circulatory troubles. There's no harm in trying.

CHAPTER 12

Many Older Folks Are Badly Nourished

DID YOU KNOW THAT, at the White House Conference on Aging in 1971, a recommendation was made for providing the equivalent of a national school lunch program for senior citizens? The reason for this is obvious. One in every ten persons alive in the USA today is over 65 years old. There are 20 million of these older folks. One million of them live in institutions, where presumably some knowledge of nutrition is involved in their meal preparation. Fourteen million live in communities with relatives or friends who may or may not know anything about preparing nourishing meals, and if they know, may or may not care enough to do it.

Five million of our older citizens live alone. These folks are probably the single most isolated group of people in our country. Says Jeanette Pelcovits in the April, 1972 issue of the *Journal of the American Dietetic Association,* "hundreds of thousands of them—even those who are mobile and could participate—live in virtual isolation, the phone does not ring, there are no visitors, there are no invitations . . . There are no incentives to action. And for the frailest, the truly physically homebound, life is lived in a kind of solitary confinement destructive to mental and physical health and humanity."

This last group is the one most likely to suffer from malnutrition, since, as just about everyone agrees, there is little incentive to prepare complete meals for just one person, little enjoyment in eating alone. As meals become skimpier, listlessness and apathy tend to make meal-preparation ever more sketchy, so the cycle goes on and on.

Dairy Council Digest for March-April, 1972 reviewed the situation in regard to the nutrition of old folks in general. "There is general consensus," it says, "that diets of elderly individuals are often nutritionally inadequate with the result that the nutritional status of some of these individuals is poor. . . . A study of nutritional status of a representative sample of aging individuals in the United States has never been made." Astonishing! Perhaps it's just that nobody cares enough.

However, nutrition studies which have been made indicate clearly that three kinds of nutritional deficiencies may be quite common in this group: anemias of various kinds, deficiencies in the water soluble vitamins B and C, and lack of calcium. "Elderly individuals of the same age vary greatly in nutritional requirements and other biological parameters," says the *Digest*.

While it is advisable to study those who make it well up into their nineties to discover what physical characteristics may be responsible for these healthy golden years, it also seems wise to consider whether those who reach seventy and beyond full of ailments, aches, pains and troubles may not possibly have excessively high requirements for many nutrients, as well as the disadvantage of eating meals which never provide enough of the essential nutriments.

The *Digest* article tells us that the condition of the mouth is an indication of nutritional health, generally speaking. Modern Westerners begin to lose teeth to periodontal (gum) disease by the time they are 40. Most experts believe that the strength of the bone in which the teeth are set has a lot to do with these problems.

In laboratory animals it has been shown that lack of calcium and phosphorus in the right proportions in the diet brings about loss of these important bones. The condition can be corrected by a diet high in calcium with phosphorus intake regulated.

When ten human patients aged 29 to 47 were given 1,000 milligrams of calcium per day in a supplement for about six months, symptoms of gum disease, including inflammation, tooth tartar and loose teeth, were reduced. X-rays showed that there was new bone formation in 7 of the ten patients. In another group of 90 patients the same calcium supplement produced the same results while another similar group, given a pill which contained no calcium, still had the same complaints.

You may wonder about the possibility of getting too much calcium. In the group of 10 described above, adding calcium supplements to the ordinary diet of these folks gave them a total daily intake of 1,200 to 1,850 milligrams of calcium. There were no adverse effects whatsoever. It is recommended, however, when calcium is increased in the diet, that zinc and magnesium should also be increased, as need for these rises when calcium intake increases.

How would one work this out in daily life? Many food supplements contain all three minerals. Foods like wheat germ, wheat bran, seeds and nuts are rich in both magnesium and zinc. Interestingly enough, in X-rays, patients who were losing teeth to gum disease were found to have the kind of bone loss in their jaws which appeared to be the forerunner of osteoporosis in later life. This is the general softening of bones which so often leads to falls and broken bones in older folks. Many nutritional experts believe that this painful disorder can be treated best with highly nourishing diets, rich in calcium, *with calcium supplements added.*

In studying anemia in older folks, doctors often find that different kinds of anemia may occur in the same individual. That is, the older person with deficiency arising from lack of iron often has, as well, that kind of anemia which occurs because of lack of vitamin B_{12} and/or folic acid. Often just the recommendation of a completely adequate diet with emphasis on the "protective" foods will bring alleviation of all these anemias. The protective foods are those which we recommend: meat, poultry, fish, eggs, dairy products, fruits and vegetables and, in the seed and cereal foods, only those which are unprocessed and unrefined—the wholegrain ones.

Pernicious anemia is a disease of older folks, almost exclusively. One theory is that they have lost the digestive juices in the stomach and the digestive "intrinsic factor" which is essential to them to absorb vitamin B_{12}, lack of which is responsible for pernicious anemia. Deficiency in folic acid "is another major cause of nutritional anemia which may be more subtle and widespread than is generally recognized", says the *Digest*. This kind of anemia may be associated with deficiency in vitamin C since both these nutrients are found in fresh fruits and vegetables.

People who do not eat enough of these foods are likely to be short on both vitamins. And of course, this includes many older folks. Fresh fruits and vegetables are expensive. You must shop often for them, for they do not keep well. The fiber they contain is hard for someone to chew, who does not have good teeth or well-fitting dentures.

All these considerations work against older folks. It's so much less trouble and expense to eat mostly those foods which we sometimes describe as "empty calorie foods" which are also almost entirely free of fiber—the sweets, the processed cereals, the cakes and cookies, the cup of sweetened tea or coffee, and so on.

Finally, the *Digest* tells us one more somber fact which

may, indeed, have a lot more to do with the sad situation of nutrition in older folks than anyone realizes. "Many drugs commonly prescribed in old age interfere with folic acid metabolism." In other words, drugs given for some condition of ill health or just as sleeping pills or tranquilizers may prevent the patient from using the folic acid, even if there is enough in his food. So everything is working against the older person. When he knows little or nothing about good nutritional practices, he is likely to make wrong choices of food more often than not.

Then, too, there is a problem of overweight. As we grow older, we tend to move around less, so we need fewer calories. But if you eliminate from your diet lots of fairly high calorie foods like meat, cheese, eggs, you are also eliminating the sources of many essential nutrients: iron, protein, B vitamins and calcium. How can you replace these and still keep weight near normal?

Obviously, the best solution is a diet which provides *only those foods which pay their way in nutrients for every calorie they contain*. "Empty calorie" foods must go. High protein foods are especially important for older folks because they must replace wornout cells. Protein is essential for this. Lean meat, lean poultry, the less fatty fish, plus eggs and milk are the essential building blocks of the good diet, no matter what your age.

Fruits and vegetables (especially the deep green leafy ones rich in iron, vitamin A and folic acid) are not worrisome for their calorie content. It's very low. Cereals should be only wholegrain ones and they should be eaten without the addition of any sugar or sugar substitute. With lots of milk or yogurt.

And why not, just as general health insurance, take every day plenty of all those vitamins and minerals mentioned above as especially likely to be lacking in the diet as we age: the B vitamins and vitamin C, calcium and iron. These are easily and inexpensively available at your health food store.

Vitamin B_{12} is not so readily available in foods, however, we list the major food source of this important B vitamin on Page 30. For the foods which contain the most folic acid, please turn to Pages 88–89. And for vegans who need to combine different high vegetable foods in order to get the right balance of amino acids, please see the chart on Page 55.

CHAPTER 13

Laughing Gas Is No Laughing Matter

NITROUS OXIDE (laughing gas) is defined this way in the latest edition of *Drugs in Current Use:* Produces analgesia and anesthesia by direct suppression of the central nervous system. Used for minor surgical procedures not requiring deep anesthesia, and for induction of surgical anesthesia, because it is more pleasant than the ether, which usually follows.

"Warnings: this gas is used with little oxygen, and the hypoxia (lack of oxygen) during anesthesia may induce serious irreversible effects on the brain. Should not be used for patients with anemia, in shock or serious circulatory defects."

To say that nitrous oxide is more "pleasant" than ether is somewhat of an understatement. As anyone knows who has been "under" nitrous oxide for dental work, the effects are more like the euphoria which a couple of alcoholic drinks seem to produce. And without any hangover.

Although nitrous oxide is very widely used for mild anesthesia, we are now beginning to discover quite serious side effects that may bring more than temporary harm. And, curiously enough, the effects appear to be related in some way to lack of vitamin B_{12}.

An article in *The Lancet* for August 12, 1978 describes the bone marrow and blood condition induced in a number of surgical patients who were given nitrous oxide during or after surgery. The authors, from St. Bartholomew's Hospital in London, England, tell us that they found earlier records of 27 patients who developed acute megaloblastic bone marrow changes in 2–14 days after admission to a hospital for severe acute illness or after undergoing major surgery. Seventeen of these had been given a half-and-half mixture of nitrous oxide and oxygen for one to eight days, we suppose to alleviate pain and produce a feeling of well being.

In all these cases the physical results *looked like pernicious anemia,* that is, a gross deficiency in vitamin B_{12}. But, strangely enough, all the patient's blood appeared to have normal levels of this B vitamin.

The doctors at St. Bartholomew set up an experiment in which they divided open heart surgery patients into three groups. The first was given the mixture of nitrous oxide and oxygen for about 24 hours, along with intramuscular injections of vitamin B_{12} before and after the operation.

A second group was given the nitrous oxide mixture only during the operation and then was given oxygen alone for the remainder of the 24-hour period. A third group was given no nitrous oxide, but got the oxygen for 24 hours.

After the operation none of the patients had lowered blood level of vitamin B_{12}. But in the second group all of the bone marrows showed the degenerative changes that are characteristic of vitamin B_{12} deficiency—that is, pernicious anemia. The first group showed the same kind of blood changes but less serious although they had been given vitamin B_{12} injections. The third group, which got no laughing gas at all, had no blood changes.

The results of the test, say the authors, suggest an abnormality of vitamin B_{12} metabolism *which is as severe as untreated Addisonian pernicious anemia*. This condition was apparent in all the patients who were given the gas and it took five days for the condition to disappear. These abnormalities were not associated with subnormal levels of vitamin B_{12} in the blood.

"Whatever the exact action of nitrous oxide," say the authors, "this study indicates that it has a definite morphological (anatomical) and biochemical effect within 24 hours. However, the abnormalities described in this paper are unlikely to explain all the cytotoxic (cell-destroying) effects of nitrous oxide and other anesthetic agents." They go on to say that this drug is useful in patients who cannot be given other anesthesia, but its value should be balanced against its possible adverse effects.

Medical Tribune for August 9, 1978 reports that "the dentist's analgesia (pain killer) commonly known as laughing gas, can cause serious neurological (nerve) abnormalities."

It seems that some dentists have been drugging themselves with nitrous oxide. The effect is so exhilarating! Five dentists were studied who had deliberately inhaled the gas regularly for periods of up to six years. And "inhalation of the gas has recently become a very widespread form of drug abuse, ... most users consider it to be a harmless high."

Here are some of the things that happen to people who are exposed often to this gas for short periods of time, or for longer periods of time. Numbness in fingers and toes. Muscle weakness. Lack of coordination. Difficulty in walking and, in some cases, impotence and loss of bladder control.

Nitrous oxide "sniffers" also report a peculiar "electric shock" sensation running from the feet up through the spinal cord to the neck.

One dentist had been in the habit of taking naps two or three times a week for several months while inhaling the gas for periods lasting from 30 minutes to two and a half hours. Because of the peculiar symptom of "electric shock", this condition was first diagnosed as multiple sclerosis. Doctors attempting to treat it also thought it might be a result of pernicious anemia (lack of vitamin B_{12}) or mercury poisoning. Dentists and other personnel in dental establishments are often exposed to toxic mercury for long periods of time when they mix the amalgam used as filling in teeth.

"The full blown picture", said Dr. Robert B. Layzer, associate professor of neurology at the University of California, "most closely resembles that of subacute degeneration of the spinal cord, but all the patients recovered slowly and steadily during abstinence from nitrous oxide."

And, perhaps most frightening of all are these facts. "An increasing number of thefts of nitrous oxide cylinders from dentists' offices and supply houses is another indication that nitrous oxide is becoming more popular as a 'recreational drug'.

"Other methods of nitrous oxide delivery include an apparatus—now promoted in underground newspapers—which allows the simultaneous inhalation of marijuana smoke and nitrous oxide."

"We feel that the toxic risks of nitrous oxide abuse need to become widely known. In thousands of dental offices there is no exhaust system for removing accumulated nitrogen oxide from the atmosphere," said Dr. Layzer.

The doctors who reported in *The Lancet* say they are sure that nitrous oxide creates a condition in which vitamin B_{12} cannot be used by the body. They don't know what it is. But apparently something about the drug blocks the entrance of the vitamin into whatever pattern of enzymes it should enter in order to preserve the health of the blood cells which are deformed in pernicious anemia. So the general effect is deficiency in vitamin B_{12}, although the blood levels remain normal.

We can probably expect a new epidemic of crippling nerve disorders in the young people using this powerful drug for "kicks". We can expect damaged brains, damaged spinal cords, damaged personalities.

If you have been accustomed to having your dental work done under the partial anesthesia which nitrous oxide produces, better think about it carefully. No one is quite certain, of course, that the damage that may be done is always completely repaired as time goes on. No one has, to our knowledge, ever studied the course of the *later* years of people who have in *earlier* years been exposed to nitrous oxide for long periods of time. It seems impossible that damage this serious could be completely repaired.

Also, it is noteworthy that the first group of patients in the London experiment—those who were given vitamin B_{12} "shots" before and after their surgery—showed less blood disorder than those who got no vitamin B_{12}. So, if you are faced with nitrous oxide exposure for whatever reason, better be sure that your blood is well fortified with vitamin B_{12}. It appears to prevent some of the damage.

CHAPTER 14

Take Care of Your Liver and Eat Liver!

YOUR LIVER is probably the most important organ in your body for the prevention of illness and the encouragement of rousing good health. It also responds to good nutrition faster and more completely than any other part of you. It has the job of tending to more body functions than any other organ. You couldn't survive a moment without it. If disease, accident or surgery destroys part of your liver, it can speedily reconstitute itself back to normal size. No other body organ can do this.

Signs of liver disorder are sometimes subtle. You are not given much warning of anything being wrong. One certain symptom of something wrong, liver-wise, is jaundice. Obstruction of the gall bladder or bile ducts can cause the yellow and green pigments of these digestive juices to accumulate and spill over into the blood. Skin turns yellow.

Malaria and some kinds of anemia destroy red blood cells. Pigments from these cells may accumulate in the liver and cause jaundice. Hepatitis and other infectious diseases may affect the liver and bring jaundice with yellowing skin.

Cirrhosis of the liver is the most serious disease which affects it. Cirrhosis causes about 20,000 deaths every year in our country. Its most common cause is alcoholism, although many people who never drink may also suffer from this disease. Some physicians believe that eating sweets is just as potent a cause of cirrhosis as drinking alcohol. In some Moslem countries where no one drinks alcohol, cirrhosis is more prevalent than in the USA. It seems possible that lack of protein and B vitamins in the diet may be responsible.

The liver is our purifier, detoxifying poisons which get into the bloodstream and excreting them before they can harm us. Even such everyday poisons as alcohol, caffeine and drugs are detoxified by the liver.

More than 500 functions have been identified for the liver. One of the most important concerns the sugar you eat. It is stored in the liver and released gradually as it is needed to supply energy for the body muscles. Eating too much sugar disorders this mechanism, for the liver has evolved over millions of years to handle only the highly diluted sugars that occur in natural foods like fruits, berries and vegetables.

The liver is also involved with body hormones. If too much of any hormone is being released from a disordered gland, the liver gets rid of the excess and excretes it, so that other glandular mechanisms will not become unbalanced. During menopause, for example, the liver maintains a good balance of sex hormones which may prevent the unpleasant symptoms of hot flashes, headaches and other circulatory discomforts.

The liver helps to digest fat and protein. It excretes the ammonia from protein foods which would otherwise accumulate and make trouble. It is involved in the process of blood clotting. It regularly "saves" the iron from red blood cells which live only a short time, and recycles it into the blood, so that we need not replenish the iron from food quite so often.

Obesity is one condition that places great strain on the liver. So is gallbladder trouble. So it is wise to avoid both these conditions. How? The same way you avoid other health problems. Stay away from those foods which produce both conditions—chiefly the refined and processed carbohydrates—everything that contains sugar and white flour, as well as highly processed supermarket cereals. See that you get plenty of protein and plenty of fibrous foods—chiefly wholegrains, wheat germ, wheat bran, rice polish, nuts, soybeans, peanuts, beans, seeds, fresh raw fruits and vegetables. These are also those foods which contain many B vitamins and minerals, which are essential for the health of the liver.

Primitive people believed that if one had a disordered body organ the best cure was to eat that organ taken from a healthy animal. And they were not far wrong. In general, we can assume that the vitamins and minerals stored in one organ of the body are there because that organ needs them to be healthy. So we can judge that the liver needs B vitamins, since animals' livers are so rich in these health-giving vitamins. We also know that the liver needs iron and copper, since these are stored in animal livers.

So, generally speaking, it is good for your liver to eat liver frequently at meals, for you are thus supplying all those nutrients, known and unknown, which keep livers healthy. The fat-soluble vitamins are stored in the liver, so any animal liver is an abundant source of vitamins A, E and K as well as the B vitamins. The liver is rich in protein, contains little fat and almost no carbohydrate. Its store of vitamin B_{12} is so large that it was originally used to cure pernicious anemia, long before scientists knew that pernicious anemia is caused by lack of vitamin B_{12}. By the same token, there may be many other nutrients in liver which we do not even know are there, which are important for preventing one disorder or another.

What about the cholesterol in liver? It does contain cholesterol, as do other organ meats and egg yolks. There is a lot of convincing evidence that cholesterol in food is not harmful and should not be avoided. Your body makes a large supply of cholesterol—in the liver, incidentally. When you eat a food containing cholesterol the liver makes less, thus keeping this fatty substance in balance. It is our belief that sugar and sugary foods cause the build-up of cholesterol in blood vessels. By avoiding sugar and sugary foods we can prevent high levels of cholesterol in the blood, as well as high levels of another fat called triglycerides.

Eat liver at least once a week. Prepare it in some way which makes it appetizing for your family. If your family does not like it or cannot eat it for some reason, then get desiccated liver and take some every day. This is whole liver with nothing but the water removed. So it contains all the liver's nutrients in concentrated form. It is available in tablets for swallowing or in powder form for mixing in food such as casseroles, soup and meatloaf.

CHAPTER 15

Vitamin B_{12} and Folic Acid Go Together

WHEN WE THINK of megavitamin therapy for mental illness, we generally think of niacin (vitamin B_3) first, then pyridoxine (vitamin B_6), then zinc, thiamine (vitamin B_1) and other B vitamins, as well as vitamin C.

Now we have valuable information from a psychiatrist who has been using megavitamin therapy for 22 years that vitamin B_{12} and folic acid are extremely valuable in treating many kinds of mental illness. And, according to Dr. L. Kotkas of Lethbridge, Canada, *they must always be used together*.

Speaking before a June, 1978 conference of the Canadian Schizophrenia Foundation, Dr. Kotkas told his audience that he has been interested in vitamin B_{12}-folic acid therapy for about 18 years. Truly a man who is years ahead of his time!

Twelve years ago, he said, while he was studying the importance of lack of absorption of vitamins, he decided to ask for routine blood counts of folic acid in all his patients.

Says he, "A large proportion varying at times between

25–50 per cent had abnormally low values, and these patients tended to be 'sicker' or more incapacitated from the psychiatric point of view." Giving these patients a combination of vitamin B_{12} and folic acid produced "dramatic improvement" in all cases which he treated in the field of depressive illness and a little less dramatic results in a wide variety of other mental conditions.

Most interesting of all, he said, is that most of these patients had normal levels of vitamin B_{12}. But the folic acid levels were below normal. When he gave them folic acid the levels of B_{12} in their blood dropped, almost as if the vitamin B_{12} had been substituting for the folic acid. And now that there was enough folic acid on hand there was no need for raised levels of B_{12}.

The two vitamins have what Dr. Kotkas calls a "tandem relationship". If B_{12} is in short supply the body will stockpile folic acid. If folic acid is in short supply, the body will stockpile vitamin B_{12}. If there is very little of one present, this interferes with the absorption of the other, so the situation becomes even more complicated.

Dr. Kotkas believes that this important relationship between the two nutrients may be the reason why some researchers have reported disappointing results when they used one or the other in treating mental illness. They simply did not understand that it's the relationship between the two that is important, so they paid no attention to providing enough of each of them, but conducted their experiments using only one.

When should these two B vitamins be used to treat mental illness, asks Dr. Kotkas. Well, he says, not just when the blood levels of these two nutrients appear to be too low. There is usually a problem of deficiency in these cases, but tests are not exact enough to depend on it.

However, he says, deficiencies in B_{12} and folic acid should be corrected *before any symptoms appear of the extremely serious anemia which is caused by such deficiency*. Rather the doctor should look for both physical and psychological signs and symptoms that seem to indicate lack of these two nutrients. Unfortunately there are no standard tests that can be given to pinpoint these symptoms.

In a deficiency of both vitamin B_{12} and folic acid you can get every psychiatric diagnostic category in the book "and a good many that aren't", says Dr. Kotkas. There is no standard, nothing regular, nothing uniform to look for, he says. However he does give some guidelines as to which conditions might be most likely to be caused by lack of these two nutrients.

1. Mental illness in the aged. "In this situation," he says, "complex inadequacies of the requirements for brain function are almost the rule in the general population". Generally old people absorb and retain B_{12} and folic acid more avidly than any other age group. "What may appear to be 'classical schizophrenia' for example when it occurs for the first time in the older age group is usually nutritional, and B_{12} and folic acid are often the key treatment".

2. So called "neurotic depressions". These are often just states of fatigue, he says, combined with anger at oneself for not being able to function as usual. In these cases, Dr. Kotkas believes, nutritional therapy is not enough and psychotherapy as well should be given with it.

3. Conditions relating to women and the female reproductive cycle, such as pregnancy, menstruation and The Pill. "A large proportion of postpartum (following childbirth) psychoses are B_{12}-folate responsive", says the Canadian psychiatrist. In other words, the depression, the crying jags, the anxiety of the new mother in many cases are due to lack of these two vitamins and can be treated by giving large enough doses of them.

4. Other gland disorders, such as underactivity of the thyroid gland and low blood sugar may also respond to this

kind of vitamin therapy, says Dr. Kotkas.

5. Conditions in which the body is absorbing large amounts of foreign chemicals in the way of alcohol, drugs, or medicines given for controlling epilepsy. Many varied manifestations of mental disorders may appear which can be treated by vitamin B_{12} and folic acid.

6. In iron deficiency anemia these two nutrients should also be given. Vitamin B_{12} and folic acid are necessary for the body to absorb enough iron, so pallor, muscle tension, myoclonus (muscle spasms), black shadows under the eyes, changes in fingernails and headaches, as well as the nervous spasms brought on by mood drugs such as the tranquilizers—all these should be expected and looked for.

Here are some of the physical signs and symptoms of deficiency conditions that can be improved by giving enough vitamin B_{12} along with folic acid.

Lack of energy and fatigue—that is, both physical and mental fatigue. One reason for this, says Kotkas, is that lack of these two vitamins produces deficiency in thiamine (vitamin B_1) *even if there is enough of this vitamin in food.* Apparently it is not absorbed well enough in the absence of the related B vitamins. "Thiamine is, of course, quite significant in fatigue states," he says.

Lethargy is another symptom and lack of volition (no ambition). Insomnia, irritability, pallor, forgetfulness, restless legs—that is, muscular cramps, twitching, sudden pains in the legs, especially at night. "Most responsive psychiatric conditions improve with intensive B_{12} and folate replacement *in from one to four days*", says the psychiatrist.

Why are these vitamins important? What do they do in terms of brain and nerve activity? First of all, both are necessary in the production of two essential substances in the brain which transmit messages along the nerves: noradrenaline and serotonin.

Two drugs can also give an effect of producing these two

essential brain substances, says Kotkas—adrenalin and amphetamine. But with these the patient gets a speedy, slightly "manic" stimulation whereas with the B vitamins there is relaxation and the improvement seems to come from within rather than being a stimulant "push" from the outside. The two drugs give a temporary euphoria—a "high"—whereas the two vitamins give instead a gentle increase in the feeling of well being. In the manic depressive patient the drugs are likely to turn the depression into fullblown mania which is very undesirable since this may result in suicide. B_{12} and folic acid are much safer, though perhaps not so dramatically stimulating.

Other differences in the way the vitamins work and the drugs work involve such things as cold hands and feet (with the drugs) plus lack of appetite, muscle tension, no proper absorption of food and so on. With the vitamins there is a stabilizing effect on circulatory and nervous symptoms—such as hot flashes in menopausal women.

Because of the difficulty in absorbing vitamin B_{12}, Dr. Kotkas usually gives it by injection. And most doctors are agreeable to giving injections of this one vitamin, we have found. In older folks especially, the digestive factor that is essential for absorbing vitamin B_{12} may be lacking in their stomachs, so they get results from injections much faster and more easily than from taking the vitamin by mouth.

Hydroxycobalamin (vitamin B_{12}) is "non-toxic in immense doses", says Kotkas, "There is no upper limit for vitamin B_{12} dosage". He says the dose he uses is about 10,000 micrograms a day. "In some cases, such as multiple sclerosis, the patients seem to need, at times, several injections a day. Usually however, the patient can clearly tell from how he is feeling how often he needs the B_{12} injections as needed. Shots are given in the morning to avoid insomnia."

He gives folic acid in doses of 10 to 20 milligrams a day and he has never seen any need for higher dosages. These are also given in the morning to avoid any stimulation that might cause insomnia if given at night.

A 1974 report in *Internal Medicine News* for February 15 relates the incidence of organic brain disorders and nerve disorders in a group of patients who were found to be deficient in folic acid, the B vitamin. These symptoms were in addition to the anemia or the alcoholism which were also present. The Yale researchers came to the conclusion that just plain folic acid deficiency can cause nerve and brain damage. A higher incidence of nerve disorders of all types was found in those alcoholics who were deficient in folic acid.

There appears to be a relationship between cyanide poisoning and the amount of vitamin B_{12} available to counteract it. According to a letter to the editor of *The Lancet* for September 15, 1973, exposure to cyanide reduces the vitamin B_{12} content of the liver which is the body's detoxifying organ.

Smokers and vegetarians have lower blood levels of vitamin B_{12} than non-smokers and non-vegetarians. Tobacco smoke contains 1,500 parts per million of cyanide. This suggests that smokers may need far more vitamin B_{12} than the rest of us to counteract the ill effects of the cyanide in the smoke. It has been recommended for many years that vegetarians assure themselves of a source of ample vitamin B_{12}, since this is almost completely absent from all foods of vegetable origin. Taking vitamin B_{12} tablets would seem best for total vegetarians, since these are made from yeast.

According to Roman J. Kutsky in *Handbook of Vitamins and Hormones*, vitamin B_{12} has a "general lack of toxicity". Relatively enormous doses have been given for a number of different disorders with no reports of any unpleasant side effects.

In general, when treating a disease with vitamin B_{12}, doctors give it by injection, since there is always the possibility that the individual may not be able to absorb it from the digestive tract. Lack of something called "the intrinsic factor" prevents absorption of this vitamin.

Much information is available on the necessity of vitamin B_{12} for older folks—especially the helpfulness of injections of B_{12} so that the problem of malabsorption is avoided. And much information on the disturbing lack of folic acid which is being increasingly found in many people, especially young women on The Pill. Now we are glad to have the information Dr. Kotkas gives us on the absolute necessity of using these two nutrients in combination at all times.

Keep this information in mind as you plan your food supplements, especially for those in the family who may be having emotional or psychological difficulties. It's the combination of the two vitamins that is important, remember. For more information on these and other vitamins, see *The Complete Home Guide to All the Vitamins* by Ruth Adams, a paperback published by Larchmont Books, in New York City. Ask for it at your health food store.

CHAPTER 16

Folic Acid, an Essential B Vitamin

FOLIC ACID IS one of the most interesting of the B group of vitamins, because of a peculiarity in its relationship with another B vitamin. It was discovered in 1941 and was named folic acid because it appears most abundantly in bright green leaves, or foliage. It was originally isolated from spinach. Never let anybody tell you that this fine dark green vegetable is not good for you! It is.

In the 37 years since its discovery, scientists have turned up an interesting complication between this vitamin and vitamin B_{12}. It seems they are closely related as we have seen. People who are suffering from a deficiency in folic acid may be helped considerably by very large doses of vitamin B_{12}. But the condition is not completely cured until folic acid is given as well.

In cases of pernicious anemia, the disease of vitamin B_{12} deficiency, the victim is often found to be suffering from a deficiency in folic acid as well. Disorders which interfere with the individual's ability to absorb food may possibly produce deficiency in both vitamins. Such disorders are sprue, celiac disease, any disorder where vomiting or diarrhea are involved. Since folic acid is thought to be manufactured, to some extent, in the healthy intestinal tract, it is believed that taking antibiotics can destroy the bacteria which do this manufacturing. So people who have been taking these drugs by mouth for long periods of time may lack these two important B vitamins.

Also there is, apparently, a very special need for folic acid in pregnancy. Some obstetricians feel women should be tested for such deficiency before they become pregnant. Many of them feel that the deficiency is widespread. Pregnant women with histories of abortion or miscarriage have been given folic acid to bring about successful childbirth.

It is especially distressing to find, in the *Journal of the American Medical Association* for October 5, 1970 an article by a Florida physician who says that folic acid deficiency has been found among women taking oral contraceptives. It appears that the drug shuts off some mechanism which is essential for them to absorb the vitamin from food. Dr. Richard R. Streiff tells us of seven women who came to his clinic with anemia. They had been taking no drugs except contraceptives which they had been taking regularly for at least 1½ years. They had been eating good diets, he says, but their bone marrow showed evidencc of megaloblastic anemia, which is the condition associated with serious lack of folic acid.

By complicated tests, this doctor discovered that the folic acid given these women in a dietary supplement was absorbed. But that form of the vitamin which appeared in food had to be processed by some body mechanism which apparently did not work when the women were taking oral contraceptives.

In another story, (*Journal of the American Medical Association,* November 30, 1970) we are told of the families of three physicians (all quite affluent) where the young daughters of the family suffered from lack of folic acid and were anemic. In every case the family was large and their eating habits were irregular, since the father had very irregular hours. Says the author, "Small families usually consume prepared meals together, whereas large families often eat food which they select as individuals or in small groups. Frequently this unsupervised diet . . . contains much carbo-

Folic Acid Content of some Common Foods
(We list micrograms per serving of 100 grams)

	Micrograms
Almonds	46
Apricots, fresh	3.6
Apricots, dried	4.7
Asparagus	89–140
Avocadoes	4–57
Barley	50
Beans, lima, fresh	10–56
Beans, lima, dry	100
Beans, Navy, dry	130
Beef, round steak	7–17
Beef, liver	290
Beef, kidney	58
Blackberries	6–18
Bread, rye	20
Bread, wheat	27
Bread, white	15
Broccoli	34
Brussels sprouts	27
Buttermilk	11
Cabbage	6–42
Cauliflower	29
Cheese, cheddar	15
Cheese, cottage	21–46
Coconut	28
Corn, sweet	9–70

hydrate, with few leafy vegetables and little protein. Since carbohydrate foods usually contain only small amounts of iron and folic acid, members of large families without organized eating habits may develop iron and folic acid deficiency." If doctors cannot discover and correct such deficiency in their own families and ferret out the reasons for it, how can they be expected to perform such a service for their patients?

Dates	25
Egg, 1 whole	5.1
Egg, yolk	13
Endive	27–63
Flour, enriched white	8.1
Flour, rye	18
Flour, whole wheat	38
Ham, smoked	7.8
Kale	50.9
Lentils, dry	99
Lettuce	4–54
Liver, beef	290
Liver chicken	380
Liver, lamb	280
Liver, pork	220
Mushrooms	14–29
Oats	23–66
Peanuts	57
Peas	5–35
Potatoes	2–130
Rice, brown	22
Spinach	49–110
Tangerines	7.4
Turnip greens	83
Watercress	48
Wheat	27–51
Zucchini	11

In the *New England Journal of Medicine* for June 9, 1966 a Connecticut physician writes to complain about the fact that folic acid is usually not in nutritional supplements given to pregnant women. He tells of three women at his clinic suffering from the megaloblastic anemia which is typical of folic acid deficiency. One of them died. She had not sought the aid of a doctor during her pregnancy. Possibly a doctor would have discovered the deficiency and could have saved her life.

Executive Health, February 1976, states that folic acid deficiency is the commonest of all vitamin or mineral deficiencies. The symptoms examined in this article certainly indicate that many of us suffer from deficiency and that some of us are at especially high risk of deficiency.

Pregnant women and women on The Pill are probably most susceptible to folic acid deficiency. Scientists have shown that if this B vitamin is omitted entirely from the diet of female rats as early as the ninth day after conception, the fetuses stop developing and are reabsorbed—that is, the mother's tissues absorb them again and they never come to birth.

If this vitamin is omitted after the 11th day, young are born, but 95 per cent of them have gross abnormalities: undeveloped organs, malformed hearts and blood vessels. Some have cataracts, some have horrible brain defects, some are born without heads.

As we reported in another chapter, Dr. Paul Newberne of Massachusetts Institute of Technology discovered that more laboratory animals deficient in vitamin B_{12} (related closely to folic acid) die from disease than animals who get plenty of these vitamins. They tested animals, giving them not quite enough folic acid and vitamin B_{12}, and found that their young were also more susceptible to disease than healthy offspring of well fed animals.

The poor nutrition of a mother during pregnancy appears

to produce some defect in her offspring which leaves them more susceptible to disease. Part of the reason seems to be abnormal thymus glands. These glands are known to have something to do with the body's susceptibility to disease.

More recent studies with human mothers show that those who are deficient in folic acid have less ability to fight off diseases. This can be overcome by giving them folic acid. So Dr. Newberne believes that many unexplained diseases of children may be the result of inadequate diet during their mother's pregnancy.

It also seems to be true, said Newberne, that animals whose mothers were deficient in folic acid when they were pregnant are more likely to succumb to cancer-causing chemicals than normal offspring.

In folic acid deficiency the red blood cells are abnormal both in size and shape. And they do not live for the expected length of time. They are produced in the bone marrow and many of them are still produced in the anemia which is brought about by folic acid deficiency. But many of them are destroyed before they begin to circulate in the bloodstream. This is what causes the kind of anemia characteristic of folic acid deficiency.

This may be mild, moderate or serious anemia. It usually produces weakness and fatigue, irritability, possibly insomnia and forgetfulness. Other quite noticeable changes are in the mouth tissues. The tongue may be sore, red, swollen, smooth and glistening. The lips and angles of the mouth may be fissured and scaly. There may be painful changes in the small intestine which can become permanent if the deficiency continues for any length of time.

Trouble with intestines means that the individual will probably not absorb other nutrients, so more deficiencies ensue. Arthritics may have anemia along with their joint pains. In some patients on whom it has been tried, folic acid has improved the anemia.

There seems to be a definite relation between lack of folic acid and mental illness, as there is with deficiency in vitamin B_{12}. Epileptic patients have shown improvement in mood and alertness when they were given folic acid. In a British study of elderly people with mental problems, almost all were found to be deficient in this B vitamin, folic acid.

There have been reports, says *Executive Health,* of improvement in non-epileptic patients with dementia after they were given folic acid. And reports of great improvement in those who were depressed and suffering from schizophrenia when they were given folic acid.

Has folic acid any relation to heart disease? It seems so. Deficiency in this B vitamin has been reported in infants and children with heart disease, both congenital and rheumatic.

There is also some evidence that lack of folic acid may be involved in the set of circumstances that bring about the initial hardening of the arteries. Seventeen elderly patients with this disorder were given 5 to 7½ milligrams of folic acid daily. Fifteen of these responded with increased blood flow through the arteries that were apparently lined with unwanted deposits. They also reported improved vision. This was supposedly due to decrease of the plaques in blood vessels leading to the retina of the eye. They also reported that they weren't so cold after taking the B vitamin, so it apparently affected the skin temperature.

In other chapters we have suggested that many older folks are anemic. Writing in the May, 1974 issue of *Geriatrics*, Dr. Thomas H. Jukes and Dr. Henry Borsook of the University of California tell us that several kinds of anemia are relatively common among older folks. Not just the usual iron deficiency anemia, but also macrocytic and megaloblastic anemia.

To prevent all three kinds of anemia, say Drs. Jukes and Borsook, we must supply five nutrients: the amino acid (fraction of protein) lysine, the B vitamins folic acid, pyridoxine (B6) and vitamin B_{12}, plus the mineral iron. And they point out, don't forget plenty of calcium, since old people tend to have osteoporosis or bone softening, which can be prevented by plenty of calcium at mealtime.

To get enough lysine, you need only a serving of meat, eggs, cheese or milk daily. Cheese is the best source of calcium—100 grams (one-fourth pound) of cheddar cheese provides the recommended 800 milligrams of calcium. For those who don't like milk, yogurt or cheese, calcium supplements are available.

Getting enough iron is a problem, Drs. Jukes and Borsook continue. If you eat enough food to get the required amount of iron, you would need 3,000 calories a day, which is far too much if you want to maintain a healthy weight. To plan a diet in which there is plenty of iron, say these two scientists, "would call for a nutritionist's knowledge of food composition and the diet would allow so little variation that it would be monotonous, and also everyone can afford a good multivitamin supplement with iron."

Vitamin B_6 is found in meat, fish, eggs, milk and cheese, wholegrain cereals and bread and soybeans.

Why should so many people be deficient in a vitamin which is readily available in so many foods? Well, many of us just don't eat those foods in which it is most abundant: liver, leafy green vegetables like watercress, spinach and broccoli. And brewers yeast which is one of the best sources.

Cooking destroys much of the folic acid in food, suggesting that we should all be eating raw green vegetables at least once a day. Boiling vegetables is especially wasteful of folic acid, since the vitamin disappears in the steam. Canning destroys most of the folic acid in foods due to the high temperatures needed for sterilization.

Then there are those conditions that render our needs for folic acid much higher. Pregnancy is one of these. The World Health Organization states that folic acid deficiency appears in one-third to one-half of all pregnant women throughout the world. And this includes American women. The Pill goes along with this deficiency, surely.

Any disease which does not allow full absorption of nutrients results in folic acid deficiency. Celiac disease, in which those foods that contain gluten cannot be eaten, causes diarrhea and changes in the intestine which interfere with absorption. Sometimes there are none of the usual symptoms of malabsorption—fatty stools, diarrhea, poor appetite, weight loss and so on.

Drugs can cause loss of folic acid—chiefly *methotrexate* which is used in the treatment of cancer and in some severe cases of psoriasis. Several drugs used to treat malaria destroy folic acid in the body. Drugs used to prevent convulsions in epileptics and others who have seizures can produce deficiency in folic acid. Folic acid and vitamin B_{12}, given together, appear to correct this deficiency.

Alcohol is the most commonly used drug which is known to deplete the body of many vitamins and minerals. Folic acid is one of these. Alcoholics taking 15 milligrams a day of folic acid were found to be absorbing the vitamin completely because, apparently, of some changes in intestinal enzymes when the B vitamin was given. It seems possible, too, that folic acid may help to prevent deleterious changes in the human liver which occur in alcoholism.

Executive Health reports that there is a strong case for *all pregnant women* to take folic acid (along with vitamin B_{12}, we would add) and to eat plenty of those foods in which it is most plentiful. Women on The Pill, invalids taking various drugs which destroy the vitamin and people who drink should also be getting plenty of folic acid, in meals and in supplements.

CHAPTER 17

Folic Acid is Related to Other B Vitamins

THERE IS A scientist at the University of California who believes that the commonest vitamin deficiency in the world is deficiency in folic acid. This affects chiefly elderly people and pregnant women, says Dr. Even Ludwig Stokstad.

Folic acid is a vitamin which is found chiefly in green leafy vegetables and organ meats like liver and kidneys. Goodly amounts of it exist also in seed foods like soybeans, lentils, nuts and whole grain cereals of all kinds. It is also believed that this vitamin is manufactured in the human intestine, although optimal conditions for this must be present or the vitamin will be lacking.

Why do we need it? Without it, we may fall prey to the symptoms of a kind of anemia which resembles pernicious anemia without the involvement of the nervous system that accompanies pernicious anemia. The patient may suffer from diarrhea, lack of absorption of food, many disorders of the digestive tract, and inflammation, burning and stinging of the mouth tissues. Folic acid will treat and cure other kinds of anemia related to pernicious anemia.

Says the *New Scientist* for September 11, 1969, "Folic acid is an essential vitamin for every living cell. It is normally in balance with vitamin B_{12} and, like it, can correct the pernicious form of anemia; but unlike it, it can produce neurological symptoms such as degeneration of the spinal cord. Professor Stokstad . . . believes folic acid deficiency to be the commonest vitamin deficiency in the world affecting particularly elderly people and pregnant women."

The problem in giving folic acid as a treatment for pernicious anemia is the matter of nerve involvement. It seems that, if the doctor gives folic acid to the pernicious anemia patient, this vitamin can cure all the symptoms of this serious disease *except the nerve symptoms*. These will progress at the same rate but the patient may be unaware of them until they have gone too far and it is too late to do anything about them. So the sensible thing appears to be to give both vitamins together, along with a substance that seems to be essential for vitamin B_{12} to be absorbed by the digestive tract.

An article in a recent issue of *Medical World News* indicates that other vitamins may be involved as well. This tells the pathetic story of a three-year-old girl, the victim of diabetes and deafness, who developed pernicious anemia at the age of 11. Vitamin B_{12} and folic acid were both given by doctors at Duke University. There was no improvement. Then a multiple-vitamin high potency capsule was given. The little girl's anemia began to improve.

After she was discharged, *she was given no more vitamins of any kind* and had a relapse. Her insulin requirements had also gone up. She was again admitted to the hospital. The doctors gave her large amounts of each of the vitamins in the multiple-vitamin capsule, until they found that large amounts of thiamine, another B vitamin, brought about fine improvement in her condition. She was sent home, again with no supplementary vitamins. Again she relapsed. This time the doctors gave her 20 milligrams of thiamine a day and sent her home telling her family to continue this treatment with thiamine. The child has had no relapses.

In the usual way of doctors, these practitioners are now trying to analyze how and why this particular vitamin made such a difference to this desperately sick child. They concluded that "she has a defect in a single thiamine-dependent enzyme and dietary amounts are insufficient to keep her from developing anemia, whereas superphysiologic amounts (that is, far more than the recommended 'normal' amounts) corrected the situation."

They do not know, they say, whether lack of thiamine had anything to do with her diabetes, her deafness or other things that were wrong with her. They fear, they say, that their treatment was too late to reverse all these conditions, for too much damage had been done.

The obvious solution, which seems never to occur to men accustomed to using vitamins as "drugs" rather than as parts of food, is to take both vitamin B_{12} and folic acid, along with a plentitude of all the other B vitamins, like thiamine, biotin, riboflavin, pyridoxine, niacin and pantothenic acid. Why not? They can't possibly harm you, in any amounts whatsoever, since they are all water soluble and do not accumulate to any degree in your tissues.

It also seems quite possible that people suffering from lack of these vitamins, and others as well, are in this condition because they have not been observing the rules of good diet all the years of their lives. Teenage girls are the worst-fed members of our society. When they become pregnant it is too late to correct all the deficiencies that exist. The last months of pregnancy appear to create a demand for much more of this vitamin, folic acid, by the unborn child.

Old folks, especially those living alone, have little interest in food and often eat only what is easiest and most convenient to buy, cook, prepare and chew. Organ meats, green leafy vegetables and whole grain cereals are not the foods generally chosen by these two groups of people.

What's the answer for preventing deficiencies of this important life-saving vitamin? First, good diet. By this we mean plenty of all the four essential groups of food: meat, fish, shellfish and poultry; vegetables (especially the green leafy ones) and fruits; dairy products and eggs, whole grain cereals, nuts and all whole seed foods like peanuts, sunflower seeds, soybeans and so on.

Then make it a habit to eat liver and/or some other organ meat at least once a week, oftener if possible. If you or other members of your family simply cannot make yourselves eat these foods, then you can get desiccated liver tablets which contain everything in the original liver except water. Take them in ample amounts. They are not drugs, but highly concentrated foods. You need plenty of them.

Finally, don't make the mistake the Duke University doctors did when they took away the little girl's vitamin pills. You, too, may have excessive need for one or more of the B vitamins, or vitamin C. Don't treat such a suggestion as unlikely. With all the drugs, chemicals and pollutants we are exposed to today which destroy vitamins, any of us is likely to have greater than "average" needs. A one-a-day vitamin of high potency is good health insurance. Taking capsules or tablets of individual vitamins is even better.

CHAPTER 18

The Great Importance of Good Nutrition in Pregnancy

SPINA BIFIDA is the name of a congenital condition which affects about two newborn children out of every thousand in our country. Medical journals call it "neural tube defect." The neural tube is the spinal column inside which is the spinal cord, the nerve center of all our movements. A newborn child may be born without complete closure of the "tube" so that part of the contents of the tube may spill out. In less serious conditions, the defect may go unnoticed until much later in life when it may cause endless back trouble for the adult.

It seems likely that some nutritional defect early in pregnancy might be responsible for such a condition, since this part of the newly conceived infant is the earliest part of the fetus to appear. So nutritional deficiency at that time would be expected to disorder the early cells which appear first in the womb.

The February 16, 1980 issue of the British medical journal *The Lancet* reported on an experiment to show, if possible, which nutrients may be the ones that are lacking in such pregnancies. The physicians from several hospitals and universities in England and Ireland cooperated in the trial. It involved 178 pregnant women who had agreed to participate and 260 women who did not wish to participate.

The nutrients selected for the test were vitamins A and D, thiamine, riboflavin, pyridoxine, niacin and folic acid (all B vitamins) and vitamin C, plus iron and calcium.

The women took the supplements for one month before conception and continued with them until after two menstrual periods had been missed, thus making certain that enough of each nutrient was available during all the earliest days of pregnancy. Women who had been taking The Pill were asked to adopt alternative methods of contraception from the time they started on the supplement, since The Pill is known to destroy several nutrients in the body.

The results were startling. Of the 178 children born to the mothers taking the supplement, only one suffered from spina bifida. Of the 260 babies born to the women who were not taking the supplement 13 imperfect children were born, with this same defect. All of the women—both supplemented and with supplements—had borne children with this defect in earlier pregnancies, so their physicians could have expected still another imperfect child. In genetic counselling clinics, the *Lancet* says, it is customary to quote the same risk in pregnancy for all mothers who have had one affected child.

A second condition which can result from the same nutritional defects in early pregnancy is *anencephaly*. This defect occurs at the top of the spinal cord rather than the bottom and it affects the brain. The brain is defective. Important parts of the brain are simply not formed.

The British doctors do not know which of the nutrients they gave their patients was the one responsible for producing the good effects. It seems likely to us that it was all of them. But folic acid seems to be the vitamin which may have had most to do with the success, since it is perhaps the one nutrient most likely to be missing in the women's diets. Folic acid is most abundant in these foods: all kinds of liver, green leafy vegetables such as spinach, salad greens and so on, wholegrains, bran and wheat germ, dried beans, lentils and peas and brewers yeast. The average British diet is probably lacking in most of these foods just as the average American diet is. There's no folic acid in hamburgers and white rolls, plus potato chips and a soft drink.

It is believed that the friendly bacteria which inhabit the intestinal tract can manufacture some folic acid, but for this the colon must be in a healthy state with friendly bacteria prevailing over those which are harmful. The "average" diet tends to create colonic conditions which discourage the growth of friendly bacteria. Mostly it is the lack of fiber in meals which brings about such a condition. People whose carbohydrate intake includes quantities of the refined carbohydrates (white sugar and white flour products along with highly processed breakfast cereals) are almost certain to have fewer numbers of the friendly colon bacteria.

It's not surprising to discover that a diet in which folic acid is lacking will also probably be lacking in most other essential nutrients. Vitamin A is most abundant in fruits and vegetables, as well as liver. Vitamin C the same. All of the B vitamins occur in largest amounts in wholegrain foods, liver, nuts, seeds, dried legumes, wheat bran and germ, as well as green leafy vegetables.

We are sorry to report that not a word is said in the *Lancet* article about giving any of the women in this experiment—either the ones who took the supplement or the ones who did not—any nutritional information which might make their next pregnancy more successful. Apparently no one sat down with each woman for a long talk about nutrition, gave them lists of foods which are the nutritious ones and lists of foods which should be avoided.

One would think that physicians who have turned up results as significant as these would think it absolutely necessary to talk to each woman about the significance of the experiment, to tell each woman that she can almost guarantee no more hideous disappointments and burdens if she will only concentrate on those foods which will adequately nourish the child she is carrying from the very moment of conception to the moment of birth.

It's obvious that any sensible woman would discover for herself how much better she feels on a diet which provides essential nutrients. She would want to continue it after her infant is born. The cost of the supplements given to the women in the experiment is minimal. Compare it to the cost of caring for a damaged child throughout a lifetime!

Other aspects of successful pregnancy which were apparently not considered in this report are: exposure to harmful environmental chemicals, smoking and drinking alcohol and large amounts of coffee or strong tea. All these have been incriminated in earlier studies of unsuccessful pregnancies. *The Lancet* does not tell us how many of the women may have been risking fetal damage by exposure to any of these risks.

Any readers who are contemplating pregnancy need to be well armed with nutritional information. Many books available at the health food store contain such information. You can obtain more by joining a group formed to combat nutritional misinformation: Society for the Protection of the Unborn Through Nutrition, (SPUN) at 17 North Wabash Avenue, Suite 503, Chicago, Ill. 60602. If you wish to make inquiries of SPUN, send along a business-sized, self-addressed stamped envelope. If you wish a copy of their very informative new booklet (10 pages) entitled *How to be a Healthy Mother and Have a Healthy Baby* put 28 cents postage on the envelope you enclose.

A New York physician reports serious possible aftereffects of deficiency in folic acid, if this occurs in a pregnant woman.

Says Dr. A. Leonard Luhby in the November, 1967 issue of *Nutrition Reviews,* folic acid deficiency in pregnant women could well constitute a public health problem "of dimensions we have not originally recognized."

We now have evidence, he says, that deficiency in this vitamin can lead to retarded growth and congenital malformations in the unborn child. Then he tells us that he found 22% of the pregnant women he examined were deficient in this vitamin. Perhaps more serious even than the mothers' lack of folic acid is the fact that babies born of such deficient mothers are themselves deficient in at least a third of the cases.

The defect can be remedied by supplements of folic acid if the lack is detected in time. There seems to be every reason to suppose that the general public, as well, is deficient in this vitamin. Unfortunately, only pregnant women are tested with this fact in mind.

We would say the findings in regard to the 55 pregnant women described by Dr. Luhby prove that individual needs for, and supplies of vitamins vary considerably. If all these women were eating the same completely nutritious diet—and the FDA insists that all Americans actually do this—then why were some of them deficient in folic acid and others not? And if some were deficient in this B vitamin, why not test them for the other vitamins as well? Isn't it probable that they lack other B vitamins, to say nothing of vitamin C, vitamins A and E?

Generally speaking, a diet which is so un-nutritious that it causes deficiencies in one vitamin is also deficient in others as well. This is because vitamins and minerals are concentrated in certain foods. Other foods contain almost none.

Anyone—and especially pregnant women—whose nutritional needs are high, who eats little of the nutritious foods and a lot of the "empty calorie" kind is probably going to be lacking in many vitamins, not just one or two.

In *Medical World News,* Dr. Myron Gordon, one of a team of pediatricians, is quoted as saying, "Some women may have a deficiency (of folic acid) for months or even years, and it should be cleared up before they have children." He believes that all his women patients should be tested for folic acid deficiency before they become pregnant. Says the *News,* "With a carefully planned diet, and vitamin supplements, adequate folic acid activity can rapidly be restored."

If these women are deficient "for years" in one important B vitamin, is it not ample indication that they have just not been eating enough of those foods which contain it? And is it not true that these same foods are the richest sources of all the other B vitamins as well? Included with the B vitamins in these valuable foods are all the minerals, fats, enzymes and other food elements that are essential for good health.

Why should American women, supposedly the best-fed women in the world, be deficient in folic acid, especially when they are young? One good reason might very well be the refining and processing of our cereal foods. Folic acid is abundant in whole grains. It is almost completely lacking in refined ones. Whole wheat flour contains 38 micrograms of folic acid; white "enriched" flour contains only 8. Wheat germ, the little nutritious nubbin which is removed from a cereal when it is refined, contains up to 160 micrograms in ¼ cup.

If these young, pregnant women have been suffering from a lack of folic acid for years, as Dr. Gordon suggests, then they have also probably been suffering from lack of pyridoxine, para-amino-benzoic-acid, choline, inositol, biotin and all the other B vitamins found in whole grain and never restored in "enriched" flour and cereal.

There is one other reason why folic acid deficiency may be so prevalent among young women. This B vitamin is quickly destroyed by sulfa drugs. These drugs may also interfere with the friendly bacteria which help to manufacture this vitamin in the digestive tract. So anyone who has been taking sulfa drugs for an infection may be deficient in folic acid and other B vitamins as well.

If you want to prevent any shortage of folic acid, better get well acquainted with those foods which contain lots of it. Make them a part of every day's meals. Since these are also the foods which are richest in all other B vitamins, including vitamin B_{12}, they are among your most valuable foods.

Physicians sometimes prescribe complete one-a-day supplements for prospective mothers and then find them developing the anemia that comes from lack of folic acid, because this vitamin is not in the supplement in sufficient amounts. One such physician wrote to the *New England Journal of Medicine,* April 7, 1966, complaining.

An article in the January, 1967 issue of *Annals of Internal Medicine* recommends as much as 200 micrograms of folic acid daily during the last three months of pregnancy. A Norwegian medical journal for July 28, 1966 recommends 500 micrograms of the B vitamin, to insure a healthy pregnancy.

The British Medical Journal, December 24, 1966, in an editorial, decided that 300 micrograms daily might be what a pregnant woman should have to insure protection against the anemia that results from lack of folic acid.

CHAPTER 19

Prospective Mothers Should Not Drink

A 160-DAY HOSPITAL TREATMENT of an alcoholic woman in a Boston hospital brought to light some significant results in terms of the effect of alcohol on folic acid.

An article in *Nutrition Reviews*, August 1979, describes this case. The article states that "anemia due to a variety of nutrient deficiencies is common in alcoholic patients. Iron deficiency anemia is found secondary to gastrointestinal bleeding. One of the major causes of macrocytic anemia in alcoholic patients is folic acid deficiency."

It seems that alcoholics are deficient in this very important B vitamin for two reasons. First, their diets almost always are deficient in the vitamin. And then the intake of alcohol blocks the formation of blood cells which is one of the functions of folic acid. So the small amount of folic acid from diet that may be available to the alcoholic cannot perform its job of keeping blood healthy because of the interference of the alcohol.

The 61-year-old waitress in Boston had lived alone for 22 years and had consumed large quantities of wine and whiskey every day for all that time. Her diet contained almost no meat, fresh vegetables and fruits. Best sources of folic acid are liver of all kinds, leafy greens like spinach and asparagus, wheat bran, legumes like lentils, beans, peas and brewers yeast. None of such food was in her diet.

The symptoms which brought this patient to the hospital were these: she was pale, had excessive urination, edema (swelling) of the ankles, was weak and breathless. She was disoriented as to time and place and she "confabulated", meaning that she rambled on and on, making no sense. She could not give the doctors any coherent account of the details of her illness.

During the time she remained in the hospital the doctors tested her reaction to diets containing no folic acid, then adding the vitamin in plentiful amounts, then giving her alcoholic drinks and testing the results on her blood cells. Results were highly significant. So long as she had no alcohol of any kind and was getting the B vitamin in a supplement, her anemia was under control, her blood cells in good shape, all the blood-forming machinery working perfectly.

As soon as she took alcohol, *with or without folic acid,* the production of blood cells declined and the anemia returned, along with iron deficiency anemia which complicated things still further.

It was clear, said the authors of this study, that in this woman, the normal formation of blood cells was inhibited even when she was getting enough folic acid for good health. When she stopped drinking alcohol and was given folic acid supplements of 75 micrograms a day, her bone marrow (where blood cells are manufactured) became normal and her red blood cells reached normal levels.

A related subject is discussed in the November 21, 1979 issue of *Medical Tribune*. Dr. Fouad Badr, of the University of Kuwait, spoke at the Third World Congress of the International Commission for the Prevention of Alcoholism and Drug Dependency.

His theme was the possibility that Down's Syndrome and

related inherited disorders may be caused by alcoholism in the parents. Dr. Badr studied chromosomes (the microscopic parts of cells that determine heredity) and found a significant increase in breakage of chromosomes in the blood of alcoholics, and also an increase in the kind of chromosomal "inversions" and translocations which occur in the blood of Down's Syndrome, Klinefelter's Syndrome and Edward's Syndrome.

The chromosome disorders are of a permanent nature, said he, meaning that the cells can reproduce, preserving the new chromosomal changes. That is, all cells produced by the originally defective cells would carry the same defects on to the next generation, and the next and the next.

He compared blood cells from 48 alcoholics with cells from 40 normal nonalcoholic controls. The average frequency of breakage was 12 times greater in the alcoholics!

It seems impossible, but at present it is true that one child in every 750 born is afflicted with Down's Syndrome. These children are mentally retarded, have characteristic facial and body structure. The disorder called "fetal alcohol syndrome" is a condition of the baby of an alcoholic mother. Here, too, the face structure is abnormal, there is mental and physical retardation similar to that of Down's Syndrome and disorders of the heart. Klinefelter's Syndrome, also mentioned by Dr. Badr, produces a child with small genital organs, excessive growth of breasts in male children and deficient chromosomes.

Edward's Syndrome brings severe mental deficiency, malformation of the hands, chest, pelvis, face and ears along with heart and kidney disorders.

The mechanism by which alcohol damages cells is not known, said Dr. Badr, but scientists do know that the damage is not done by the alcohol itself but by one of the breakdown products called acetaldehyde. He believes that the tragic condition of babies born to alcoholic mothers may not be entirely due to chromosome breakage. It's quite possible that the pregnant woman who drinks heavily while she is pregnant has been drinking for a long time before she became pregnant.

In any event, the damage is done by drinking. It seems quite possible, too, that not all such defective babies are the result of alcoholism. Undoubtedly the mother's age plays a part in the birth of a Downs' Syndrome child. And we haven't a doubt that many of the environmental pollutants to which we are all exposed every day have genetic consequences which have not been investigated up to now, and which may be responsible for many of these damaged children.

We are told that alcoholism is a problem of increasing concern in schools and colleges these days. The prospect of many teenage girls becoming alcoholics in school and then continuing to drink while they bear children is a grave threat not only to the happiness and stability of the women's lives, but also to the welfare of the rest of us who will eventually be burdened with the care of both the alcoholics and their imperfect children.

The authors of the *Nutrition Reviews* material concluded their article with the words, "The interaction of (alcohol) metabolism with the folate (folic acid) cycle is more evidence for a two-fold approach to the rehabilitation of alcoholic patients. Eat well and stop drinking."

If you are interested in further information on alcoholism in pregnant women in relation to the unborn child, write to Wisconsin Clearinghouse for Alcohol and Other Drug Information, University of Wisconsin Hospital and Clinics, 1954 East Washington Ave., Madison, Wisconsin 53704. Ask for their list of publications. Send along a self-addressed, stamped envelope.

CHAPTER 20

Folic Acid and Your Sex Life

SOME YEARS AGO a physician experimented on himself to find out whether folic acid can be manufactured in the human intestine or whether it must be obtained in food. Dr. Victor Herbert, then at Boston City Hospital, put himself on a diet from which all folic acid was removed. He did this by boiling all his food three times. The heat and moisture involved in this process virtually destroyed not only all the folic acid but most other vitamins as well.

Then he took plenty of all other vitamins in a capsule, so that any nutritional difficulties he encountered would be certain to arise from folic acid deficiency. They began very soon. After three weeks the level of folic acid in his blood was low. At the end of seven weeks the first signs of abnormality in his blood appeared. After he had been on the deficient diet for 16 weeks, he became sleepless, forgetful and increasingly irritable. He lost weight. By the nineteenth week his bone marrow showed unmistakable changes in the cells, indicating absence of folic acid.

He took some folic acid in a tablet. Within 48 hours his bone marrow tests returned to normal, his mental symptoms cleared up. He believes that this test proves that human beings must get folic acid in their meals or they will eventually develop the perhaps fatal anemia that characterizes this deficiency. Not many of us boil our food three times in an effort to induce a deficiency of folic acid. But, as you think over the diets of your friends and neighbors, perhaps you have observed some which qualify as diets very low in folic acid. The vitamin is easily destroyed by both boiling and sunlight.

Other symptoms of the anemia which occurs when folic acid is lacking are these: weakness, loss of appetite, diminished vigor. Also digestive disturbance—flatulence, impaired absorption of food, and diarrhea. Skin and tissues of the mouth, gums, tongue and eyes are pale. Eventually there is breathlessness, fatigue and, because of the reduced number of oxygen-carrying red blood cells, heart damage and eventual death. A little dose of folic acid can end all these symptoms very quickly.

Alcoholics suffer from deficiency in folic acid. In some startling experiments, Dr. Herbert and a colleague tested alcoholic patients by giving them a few drinks in the hospital. First they cured the anemia of the alcoholics, then they gave them daily doses of alcoholic drinks. Within 10 days the bone marrow symptoms of folic acid deficiency appeared again.

The physicians gave folic acid. It did no good, so long as the men went on drinking. By discontinuing the alcohol or by giving *very large* doses of folic acid the physicians could prevent the anemia from returning. They finally got to the point where they could tell exactly how much alcohol every day would result in severe impairment of bone marrow. They believe that one reason alcoholics improve in a hospital is that alcohol is unavailable and folic acid *is* available in the hospital diet.

Arthritis patients have been found to be lacking in folic acid. Diets that are not nourishing, increased need for folic acid because of the arthritis or possibly increased demand because of the aspirin taken by the patient may be reasons for this. No one knows. Patients with many kinds of skin disorders are also found to be deficient in folic acid.

But pregnant women are most likely to show this deficiency. Apparently the unborn child uses up whatever folic acid is available in the mother and the health of the mother suffers. We are told that studies of folic acid lack in pregnancy may explain many cases of "spontaneous" abortions, miscarriages and hemorrhaging in pregnancy. No one is certain whether the deficiency in folic acid is only one part of a disturbed state of health or whether it is the folic acid deficiency that directly triggers the health disasters.

One London physician stated that about 60 per cent of all pregnant women are unable to meet the demands for folic acid in pregnancy. He based his conclusions on studies of 154 pregnant women. Those who were also deficient in iron suffered the most. The iron deficiency sometimes concealed the lack of folic acid. Sometimes giving folic acid prevented both deficiencies. The pregnant women's anemias responded quickly to injections of folic acid given every other day for six doses.

By 1969 the *Journal of the American Medical Association* was printing articles on folic acid deficiency in women on The Pill. By 1973 the *Journal* reported megaloblastic changes in women on The Pill in the lining of the cervix, similar to those found in folic acid deficiency. Nineteen per cent of 115 women taking The Pill had these symptoms—of "severe" folic acid deficiency. Such changes were not observed in other women on the Pill. Examining the blood of these women did not disclose any apparent deficiency. It seemed to be localized in the tissues of the cervical area.

The authors of the *Journal* article point out that changes such as they found in the cervix of their patients are sometimes mistaken by doctors for pre-cancerous changes. But just giving folic acid repaired the damage in a short time. Seventeen to 21 per cent of their patients had low levels of folic acid in their blood, but, they say, women who do not have these typical stigmata also have low levels of folic acid in their blood.

They say that there are strong associations between folic acid and sex hormones. It's possible, they say, that oral contraceptives act to cause the body to use up its store of folic acid more rapidly and this is why so many women taking The Pill are short on this important B vitamin. Women who get serious anemia from the folic acid lack following The Pill may be extreme instances of a body condition which is apparently much more prevalent when it is localized in the cervix.

The Lancet for April 14, 1973 tells us that infants have far greater need for folic acid than adults. Premature babies are thought to need about 10 times more folic acid than adults. So early childhood is a time when folic acid deficiencies are very likely to show up, says the *Lancet* editorial. Premature babies tend to develop megaloblastic anemia when they are from six to eight weeks old. Perhaps they should be getting this B vitamin routinely, say the authors.

Other children are also at risk from this kind of deficiency. Babies who develop digestive problems, pneumonia or some other infection, those who have iron deficiency anemia, or scurvy or conditions of malnutrition are more apt to suffer, too, from folic acid lack. They point out that an exclusive diet of goat's milk may produce such a condition since goat's milk has less folic acid than cow's milk. Children on special diets, those with diseases that reduce their appetites or their absorption of food, or diseases which increase their need for folic acid—all these may show evidence of deficiency.

Here are some conditions that produce such deficiency: sickle-cell anemia, *thalassemia major*, hereditary *spherocytosis*, and celiac disease. Testing for folic acid deficiency is a good test for celiac disease. Epileptics taking anti-convulsant drugs are also at high risk when it comes to folic acid. Heart disease in children may produce folic acid deficiency. Congenital or rheumatic heart disease are two of such conditions in which deficiency is often found. Apparently low levels of folic acid may harm the brain, so it is wise to discover the deficiency early and give the vitamin, say the authors.

The amount of folic acid you could get in a food supplement was once limited by the FDA because of a peculiar quirk in its relationship to vitamin B_{12}. Lack of either of these vitamins produces a similar kind of anemia. The anemia caused by lack of vitamin B_{12} produces some serious nerve symptoms which are not caused by lack of folic acid. So if the doctor apparently cures the anemia by giving folic acid, a deficiency in vitamin B_{12} may still continue and destroy nerve tissues before it is discovered. It seems obvious that the best way to prevent this *is to supply supplements which contain both vitamins*. But the easy, practical way is never the way the doctors and the FDA decide to do things.

So the only answer is to make sure you are getting enough of both vitamins along with all the other vitamins of the B complex or group. Foods richest in folic acid are these: Liver, first and foremost. It contains three or four times more folic acid than any other food. Give it to your family at least once a week, oftener if possible. If they refuse to eat it, devise original ways of preparing or camouflaging it so they will enjoy it. Or give them desiccated liver tablets.

The second most abundant source of folic acid is yeast—brewer's yeast. In many of the experiments described in literature about folic acid, yeast extract was given as the sole source of folic acid and successfully prevented deficiency. Get your brewer's yeast at the health food store.

Other good sources are wheat bran, wholegrain cereals and green leafy vegetables of all kinds. Best among these are the dark green ones—spinach, kale, escarole, turnip greens, watercress and so on. Asparagus and cucumbers, cauliflower, cabbage, broccoli and beans of all kinds are good sources. Cottage cheese contains folic acid.

One final note. Breast feeding, surely the best way to feed infants, can easily prevent folic acid deficiency in the baby only if the mother's diet has provided enough folic acid. One mother was reported who lost three breast-fed babies to megaloblastic anemia. The fourth developed anemia at 14 weeks. The mother was given plenty of folic acid during her next four pregnancies and had four more healthy children.

CHAPTER 21

Folic Acid Deficiency in Crohn's Disease

DIGESTIVE DISEASES ARE ignored or underestimated by the public, the medical profession and the government, stated a recent report by the newly formed National. Comission of Digestive Diseases, according to *Medical World News* for January 2, 1980.

Under a mandate from Congress, this commission studied the situation and issued a report containing 23 specific recommendations for federal action to combat the problem. Up to now there has been almost no response from Congress, although doctors appear to be a bit concerned about the problem.

One of the Commission's recommendations was a grant of $58 million "for digestive diseases." This would include an information clearing house, funding for digestive disease instruction in medical schools and an advisory board to monitor the progress of the commission's recommendations.

It seems the commission found that medical schools teach almost nothing about digestive diseases. Fewer than one per cent of medical faculty members are experts in gastroenterology (study of the stomach and digestive tract). One-third of the medical school pediatrics departments do not even have a pediatric gastroenterologist on the faculty. So, many physicians know almost nothing about the subject.

This is probably one of the reasons why digestive diseases account for 10 per cent of health expenditures and 10 per cent of all deaths in our country, ranking third as a cause of death.

One probable reason for the apparent unconcern of the medical schools about digestive diseases is that they have been brainwashed into believing that the American diet is perfect. Since food, beverages and drugs are the only things that go into the digestive tract, therefore, the reasoning seems to be, digestive diseases must fall from heaven upon certain people for no reason at all. The idea of inquiring about the patient's diet and possibly changing it for the better never seems to occur to the average physician.

Take Crohn's Disease, for example. This is a disorder of the small bowel, and sometimes of the large bowel, which brings about abdominal cramps, chronic diarrhea, frequent bloody stools with mild fever, lack of appetite and weight loss. There may be what doctors call "an abdominal mass" in the abdomen.

As might be expected, many nutritional deficiencies result when diarrhea persists for any length of time. So it should not be surprising to find that victims of this disorder (also called *regional enteritis* or *terminal enteritis*) may be deficient in vitamins and other substances.

In the same issue of *Medical World News* appears an article on treating Crohn's Disease with total intravenous feeding. That is, the patient eats nothing. Tubes supply daily nutrients of protein, carbohydrate, fat, vitamins and minerals. This is to "rest the bowel." Crohn's Disease afflicts an estimated one million to two million people in our country.

A University of Chicago specialist estimates that one fourth to 60 per cent of all Crohn's Disease patients will have to have surgery eventually. That is, the affected parts of the intestines will be removed.

Considering that medical schools teach almost nothing about digestive diseases, and less than nothing about nutrition, it follows that medical practice finds that the best means of control is feeding the patient artificial food through a tube in the arm, and finally cutting away all inoperative parts of the intestine. The kind of food being eaten by the patient is somehow never suspected as the cause of the disease. *Why not?*

Obviously, the human intestine evolved throughout the past ages to deal successfully and healthfully with a certain kind and quality of food—the kind and quality of food that would nourish a vast population of helpful bacteria in the colon which would keep this part of the digestive tract healthy.

What has happened to upset this perfectly functioning operation? First of all, practically all the fiber has been removed from the average American diet. An excretory tract which evolved to handle large amounts of fiber is unable to make the transition to fiberless food in the brief space of time since refined carbohydrates appeared on the scene. They are all but totally bereft of fiber and they make up about one-half of the average American diet.

Up until a hundred years ago most people were eating lots of raw fruits and vegetables plus wholegrains, along with seeds and nuts (all rich in essential fiber) as a major part of their meals. Bread was tough and chewy, loaded with the fiber of bran and germ which has been carefully removed from bread and cereals in the past 50 years or so.

Sugar, derived from a tough, thick stalk of grass, has been refined into a fine white powder, devoid of any nutrients except carbohydrate. Such a food does not exist in nature. Human beings have created it. And today most Americans are eating two pounds of sugar a week or more. According to studies by Dr. Alexander G. Schauss and his colleagues at the Institute for Biosocial Research, Tacoma, Wash., some juvenile offenders were found to be eating between 274 and 465 pounds of sugar a year in candy, soft drinks and other junk foods.

Even up to 75 years ago sugar was a delicacy used by the teaspoon for flavoring, as one uses spices. It was expensive and hard to get. Today it is one of the least expensive grocery items and it is present, unseen, in practically every food in the supermarket except those that have had no processing of any kind—fresh fruits and vegetables, real wholegrains, nuts, seeds, dairy products, meats, eggs, fish and poultry. This is the reason we urge our readers to buy only these fresh, unprocessed foods and make meals "from scratch" at home.

But recent disclosures in regard to the essential nature of fiber in foods may be bringing about a change in medical thinking. Of course, it may take another 50 years before the news leaks down to all physicians but some mighty convincing evidence is even now appearing in leading medical journals. About Crohn's Disease for example.

The *British Medical Journal*, Volume 2, 762, 1979, reported that a survey of a large number of victims of Crohn's Disease showed that they were eating far more sugar, far less fiber and fewer raw fruits and vegetables than healthy matched controls.

"It might be argued," said the researchers, "that patients (with Crohn's Disease) may gradually modify their diets in the months and years before their symptoms become troublesome, eating more sugar to try and counteract weight loss or lassitude and eating less raw food to counteract loose stools." But the scientists found, they said, that this was not the case. There was no difference between patients with recent and long-lasting symptoms so far as their consumption of sugar was concerned, as well as raw fruits and vegetables.

So the doctors decided to try a high fiber diet for patients with Crohn's disease. They put 32 patients on a diet rich in fiber and totally lacking in refined carbohydrates (that is, sugar and everything made from it, as well as processed white flour and cereals.) They compared results over almost five years with results in other Crohn's Disease patients eating the usual diet prescribed for these cases—with almost no fiber and no restrictions on refined carbohydrates.

At the end of this test, they found that the individuals on the fiber-rich diet spent only 111 days in the hospital compared to 533 days in the hospital for those on the low fiber diet. Only one of the fiber-diet patients needed any surgery (and in him the necessity for surgery was noted before the diet was begun). Five of the patients on the low fiber diet had to have bowel operations.

Say the authors of this report in the highly respected *British Medical Journal*, "In our experience with this diet, which totals 150 patient-years, no patient has suffered intestinal obstruction, though many originally had intestinal strictures." Just the same, they recommend that their patients add fiber *gradually* to their diets and chew their food well to prevent any large, tough pieces of food getting into these damaged colons.

What's the answer for the millions of Americans who suffer from this debilitating and unpleasant disease with its almost certain termination in drastic surgery? There seems to be no reason to hesitate in beginning gradually to add fiber to your diet. If your doctor has been prescribing a low-fiber diet and is horrified at the thought of putting fiber-rich foods into a diseased intestinal tract, suggest that he read the article in the *British Medical Journal*. The hospital library has this publication on its shelves.

The easiest and least expensive source of fiber is bran—plain, unprocessed miller's bran available at your health food store. It's best probably to start with a fine grind rather than a coarse one. Add one teaspoon to your breakfast cereal or your luncheon soup or your dinner salad. It's best to soak the bran for a few minutes in milk or some other fluid. Gradually add a bit more bran every day and note the results. You may have a brief few weeks of increased gas and perhaps some other distressing symptoms. But these will improve rapidly. As you proceed to add bran, along with fresh raw fruits and vegetables to your meals, you are almost bound to find that the diarrhea slackens and finally disappears as you gradually change your diet into the kind your ancestors ate while human digestive tracts were evolving. Of course, an important part of the treatment is to eliminate sugar and everything that contains it.

Since helpful colon bacteria are essential to a well functioning excretory tract, it would also be helpful to add every day some yogurt or other source of the Lactobacillus bacteria which do such a good job of maintaining the health of the entire excretory tract.

Lack of the trace mineral zinc may be one reason for some of the complications of Crohn's Disease, such as dermatitis, lack of appetite, growth retardation in young people and undeveloped sex organs. It seems reasonable to assume that all the trace minerals and many minerals needed in larger amounts would be lacking in an individual whose chronic diarrhea makes absorption of these nutrients impossible. So adding supplements of trace minerals, especially zinc, would probably help in improving the condition of Crohn's Disease. A diet rich in fiber, especially bran and wheat germ, would, of course add considerable zinc to meals.

An article in the *British Medical Journal,* April 13, 1968 reported on 64 patients suffering from Crohn's Disease. Doctors found that most of them were lacking in folic acid. Vitamin B_{12} is so closely related to folic acid that the London doctors first had to make sure that none of the symptoms they found were caused by lack of vitamin B_{12}. Only one patient proved to be lacking in this vitamin.

The rest were sorely deficient in folic acid. The authors

say this may be due to a combination of inadequate intake of the vitamin, excessive needs for the vitamin and/or lack of absorption of the vitamin.

It is concluded, say the authors, that severe deficiency in folic acid is a frequent complication of Crohn's Disease and that giving the B vitamin may prove beneficial in a high proportion of such patients. They reminded their physician readers that vitamin B_{12} deficiency is so common in people with Crohn's Disease that they should be certain to exclude deficiency in this vitamin before deciding that there is a folic acid deficiency.

It is absolutely essential for all of us, those who are ill from some disease which prevents absorption of nutrients and those of us who are healthy, to remember that these two vitamins should always be considered together and should not be taken in large amounts apart from one another. If you are taking one, always be sure that you are also getting plenty of the other.

An example of what can happen is the story told in the *New England Journal of Medicine* for November 15, 1973. A 48-year-old Canadian began to suffer from lack of appetite and fatigue and became gradually weak and pale. He had some dizziness and nausea and noticed that his ankles were swollen. And he became depressed.

On the advice of a friend, he took some supplements of folic acid—containing eight milligrams of the vitamin daily. He began to feel better at once and almost cancelled the appointment he had made with his doctor. But he decided to keep it. The doctor gave him tests for many different conditions and found that he was very deficient in vitamin B_{12}.

The large doses of folic acid had cured some of the symptoms of the anemia of which he was suffering, but had not cured others. If he had not gone to his doctor and gotten a test, he might have continued to develop an extremely serious condition as a result of vitamin B_{12} anemia—pernicious anemia. This condition causes degeneration of the spinal cord with many serious, perhaps fatal complications in nerve health.

There is no suggestion that the folic acid, taken in context with other B vitamins, is harmful. It cures completely the condition that results from folic acid deficiency. But it cures it so completely that symptoms of vitamin B_{12} deficiency are masked, as they were in this case, and the nerve disorders proceed without the individual being aware that his nerves are gradually being harmed.

The Canadian doctors gave their patient injections of vitamin B_{12} and he returned to good health speedily.

The Lancet for January 10, 1970 reported on a test for toxicity of folic acid. Fourteen healthy volunteers were given large doses of this B vitamin (15 milligrams daily) to see what would happen to the vitamin B_{12} state they were in. The test had to be stopped after one month because the volunteers developed very disturbing symptoms—mental changes, sleep disturbances and digestive disorders.

Handbook of Vitamins and Hormones by Roman J. Kutsky reports "No toxicity" in human beings no matter how high the dosage of folic acid. So perhaps the symptoms experienced by the British volunteers were symptoms of imbalance between this B vitamin and its closely associated vitamin—B_{12}.

Whatever the explanation, it is well to keep in mind that it is always unwise to take large doses of folic acid without being certain that you are getting enough of vitamin B_{12}.

CHAPTER 22

Older Folks Are More At Risk Nutritionally Than the Rest of Us

ONCE AGAIN A clarion call has been sounded on the importance of good nutrition to our older citizens and the price we pay in health services when we neglect them, and especially when we neglect their nutritional state.

In *The Journal of the American Geriatrics Society* for August, 1973, Dr. Dodda B. Rao of Oak Forest Hospital, Oak Forest, Illinois, writes on the problem of nutrition in the aged. It is a very practical and thorough treatment of the subject, part of Dr. Rao's doctoral thesis.

Says Dr. Rao, "Increasingly recognized is the conspicuous lack of appropriate concern and action by both professional and political powers for the many needs of the aged population. The extent of hardship and unmet needs continues to mount, even in an affluent society. Indeed, the 'invisibility' of these unfortunate citizens is paving the way for them to emerge as the ''new poor'." And "Nutritionists have never been able to define accurately the nutritional needs for the elderly."

There are four conditions that may bring about malnutrition in the aged, according to Dr. Rao: Undernutrition which means just plain not getting enough food; overnutrition which means getting too much of the wrong kind of food; a specific deficiency in some one or several individual nutrients and, finally, an imbalance which results from a disproportion among the essential nutrients—let's say, too much carbohydrate and fat in proportion to the amount of protein in the diet which is a fairly common failing in inadequate diets in our country.

And what are some of the reasons why malnutrition is widespread—and probably becoming more so as years go on?

1. Limited income may make it impossible for the older person to buy the right food, cook it and refrigerate it.

2. He or she may lack appetite due to loneliness, unhappiness or bereavement. Even if one's immediate family is intact, by the time one reaches the age of retirement many of one's friends have died. And as we grow older, deaths of close friends become more common.

3. Reduced physical activity and increased fatigue or weakness may bring about lack of interest in preparing meals, so they become less and less nutritious and well balanced.

4. Elderly people living alone become isolated, especially those who live in cities. From plain lack of social contact they may degenerate physically and mentally.

5. Deprived of the support of family, friends or community, they may become apathetic, depressed and lack appetite.

6. Chronic alcoholism plays a role in old age, as at the other times of life. And many old people follow fads and limit their eating accordingly.

7. If they suffer from some chronic disease, they may

lack appetite.

8. Bad teeth, poorly fitting or missing dentures may influence their eating habits greatly.

9. If they are confused or depressed (and many old people are and part of the reason is undoubtedly malnutrition), their eating habits and hence nutritional health may suffer even more.

10. A combination of several or all of these factors may be responsible for malnutrition among the elderly. In addition most people accumulate food habits as they age. By the time they are really old, many people are "set in their ways" and almost nothing else in life can exert as much tyranny over one's meals as eating habits which are determined early in life and never changed.

Dr. Rao explains just how it is so difficult to determine how and where any older person is suffering from malnutrition. In the absence of severe malnutrition, Dr. Rao says, it is difficult to assess the nutritional state of the older person. (We would suggest that one reason it is so difficult is that few physicians are capable of making such an assessment because they have learned so little about nutrition during their years in medical school.)

For example, glossitis (inflammation of the tongue) may be caused by lack of niacin (B_3), folic acid, riboflavin (B_2) or vitamin B_{12}. Uremia may bring about this condition. Antibiotic drugs given for long periods of time can produce it. So if the older person has glossitis which of the above is responsible?

Angular stomatitis is inflammation of the corners of the mouth. It may mean that the patient has been getting too little riboflavin, niacin or pyridoxine (vitamin B_6). It may mean just that his dentures fit badly. Wearing dentures may bring about many different changes in tongue and gums that cannot be distinguished from the destruction wrought by vitamin deficiency. Poor oral hygiene or gum disease may do the same.

"Most signs of malnutrition are not specific for lack of any one nutrient," says Dr. Rao. "They even can be produced by a combination of various non-nutritional factors." And doctors don't really understand much about the whole subject. We would point out, for the benefit of anybody who suffers from any of the above confusing symptoms, that it is certainly not necessary for a doctor to examine you and tell you that you may or may not be suffering from vitamin deficiency, in order for that deficiency to be corrected. *You can certainly correct it yourself.* Especially with the B vitamins and vitamin C you are perfectly safe in taking even very large doses of these nutrients. If the symptom disappears six months or so after you begin an intensive course in vitamin and mineral therapy along with good diet, then it's pretty obvious that it was not caused by poorly fitting or missing teeth, or gum disease or drugs you might be taking. It was caused by nutritional deficiency and you corrected it wisely and conservatively all by yourself!

It astonishes us that any physician, treating an elderly person would not prescribe potent vitamin and mineral supplements, whether or not he thinks the current symptoms may be due to deficiency. Why take a chance? Why not just use the supplements along with whatever other treatment seems to be necessary? Why not utilize any possible treatment that may help—and surely nutritional supplementation is one beneficial and inexpensive treatment.

A lot of us do not have good eating habits, says Dr. Rao. And "most problems of the aged are compounded by poor nutrition. Nutritional deficiencies respond well to treatment, with dramatic improvement in comfort, strength and efficiency. This, in turn, enhances psychologic well-being. *Total rehabilitation is unattainable without nutritional rehabilitation.* With good nutrition, the person is better equipped physically and emotionally to enjoy his added years." Amen.

What is an ideal food for elderly people, Dr. Rao asks, which will meet all their needs nutritionally and practically? It must be acceptable to them and readily available. It must be cheap and easily prepared, using the ingredients one might have on hand—nothing exotic. It must be easy to prepare quickly, appetizing and easy to chew and digest. It must keep well under inadequate conditions of storage. It must be amenable to being used in liquid form if necessary, easy to mix with other foods and rich in protein, minerals, vitamins and calories.

Let's list some nutritious foods and see how they qualify. Eggs come to mind first. You can prepare them in hundreds of ways—all of them easy and fast. They are easily chewed and digest probably better than any other food. They can be made into eggnogs. And they are more nearly the "perfect" food than any other, in terms of essential nutrients. They lack nothing but vitamin C.

Milk and meat also qualify except that they too must be constantly refrigerated.

Wholegrain cereals from the health food store are perhaps the most nourishing foods of vegetable origin which meet every criterion listed above and they can be stored for appreciable lengths of time—at least as long as it takes to eat your way through a full carton or jar. Wheat germ is the most highly nutritious of such foods. If it is bought in small quantities it does not need refrigeration, although it is preferable to refrigerate it always.

Fruit juices, bottled or canned, provide vitamin C, vitamin A and many minerals, as well as healthful natural sugar. They can be used over cereal, as desserts, as beverages, as snacks. Nuts and dried fruits are highly concentrated sources of nutrients: protein, B vitamins and minerals, in the case of nuts, and natural sugars and minerals in the case of dried fruits. They present problems of chewing for people with poor or missing teeth. But a blender can solve such problems.

Nuts and dried fruits can be whizzed into desserts, beverages, sauces or butters. Peanut butter, almond butter and tahini are excellent and highly nutritious foods, all easily available at your health food store.

The trap into which so many old people fall is precisely the same trap that threatens us all in a society where packaged and boxed goodies are arranged in block-long shelves in the supermarket, with no indication given as to how nutritious a food each box contains or how expensive it is *in terms of protein, vitamins and minerals*.

This is why it is always best to buy in the supermarket only foods that are not boxed, hence not processed or refined or chemicalized. Buy meat, fish, poultry, eggs, dairy products, fresh fruit and vegetables and you can't go wrong in a supermarket. For your staple foods, visit the health food store, for only there can you find whole foods, not processed, not refined, not prettied up with pounds of chemical additives and dyes. Whether you are counted among the older generation or whether you buy food for a young family, these are the best rules to follow.

CHAPTER 23

A Folic Acid Deficiency May Develop as We Age

"SOME VITAMIN DEFICIENCY is almost universal in hospitalized populations in the USA, especially among older persons," say three physicians from the New Jersey Medical School in an article in the *Journal of the American Geriatrics Society*. "Deficits among the elderly may be more widespread than a few surveys have revealed. Long-term effects of subclinical malnutrition may be cumulatively injurious to the aged."

The three physicians mention the following nutrients as those most likely to be short in the diets of elderly people: vitamin B_6 (pyridoxine), vitamin B_{12}, vitamin C, vitamin B_1 (thiamine) and folic acid. Not getting enough iron may decrease absorption of folic acid and vitamin B_{12}, thus making a bad situation worse. Analyses of the blood indicate that elderly folks are likely to have low levels of vitamin C, thiamine, vitamin B_{12}, folic acid and panthothenic acid (another B vitamin). These apparently decline with age, though the reasons for this are not clear. Evidence indicates that older people have less hydrochloric acid in the stomach, as well as fewer digestive enzymes. These are necessary for absorption of nutrients. Sluggish livers and bile tracts may be partly responsible, since these are involved with absorption of fats, including fat soluble vitamins like A and E. This brings about a disordered condition of the lining and muscles of the intestines which makes poor absorption more likely.

Deficiency in folic acid is common in the elderly, say the authors. In one study 40 per cent of the older folks examined had low blood levels of this B vitamin—and had, as a result, the anemia which is characteristic of this deficiency. In some of these people it was obvious that just not getting enough foods rich in folic acid was the reason for the deficiency. But in other studies of hospitalized people, the diet appeared to contain plenty of folic acid, but it was just not being absorbed by these older people. So there appears to be no doubt that, in some older folks at least, even a fair amount of folic acid in a good diet is not absorbed, so they still develop anemia because of this.

The three doctors set up an experiment to test their theory. They assembled a group of 12 young, healthy volunteers and 24 elderly volunteers, from 73 to 101 years of age. They gave them all the same supplements: vitamin B_2 (riboflavin), vitamin B_6 (pyridoxine) pantothenic acid (another B vitamin) and folic acid. All the vitamins were from brewers yeast, which is an excellent source of all B vitamins.

Both young and old successfully absorbed the first three vitamins, and the young people absorbed the folic acid. But the older folks did not. This seemed to indicate what the doctors had expected—that older folks do not absorb folic acid very well from natural food sources, for, of course, the folic acid in yeast is in a natural state.

Then the doctors gave *synthetic* folic acid to their elderly volunteers and the folic acid levels in their blood increased at once. It seems that the digestive mechanisms which were not functioning well in the elderly people were not necessary for them to absorb the synthetic form of the vitamin. It was almost as if the vitamin had been injected instead of being taken by mouth.

We know that doctors often inject vitamin B_{12} in their patients (especially older folks) who have lost the ability to absorb it from the digestive tract. Now it appears that a synthetic form of folic acid taken by mouth may answer the same purpose in regard to this B vitamin. The New Jersey authors suggest that vitamin B_{12} should be given at the same time as the folic acid for these two vitamins have a peculiar relationship which makes this advisable. Both vitamins can be used to treat pernicious anemia. But giving folic acid alone may clear up most of the symptoms of this very serious form of anemia while not affecting the nerve symptoms. So the nerve symptoms may progress and become extremely serious or even fatal before the cause is apparent.

For this reason it is always best to take the two vitamins together, never separately, in large amounts. And large amounts are apparently necessary for elderly people when it comes to folic acid. Smaller doses than 25 to 50 micrograms are not absorbed by older folks, say the doctors. And a diet which appears to be nutritionally adequate in every respect, including folic acid, may not prevent a quite serious anemia in elderly people unless they get at the same time some folic acid in synthetic form—that is, not as folic acid appears in food. The synthetic kind of folic acid can apparently bypass the defective digestive apparatus and get into the blood satisfactorily.

Possibly the most discouraging aspect of this story is that the less folic acid you absorb the worse the condition of your digestive tract becomes, so that, as time goes on, you will undoubtedly absorb less and less of this important vitamin. So it's a vicious cycle. And the folic acid deficiency becomes worse and worse as time goes on.

Folic acid is not the easiest vitamin to get in abundance even in a fairly well planned diet. The diet of tea and toast so common to elderly recluses contains almost none. Best sources of this B vitamin are liver (of course), wholegrain breads and cereals, legumes of all kinds (like lentils and peanuts), and green leafy vegetables like spinach, watercress and kale. Most American diets are not especially rich in such foods and, we suspect, the diets of most elderly people contain even less than the diets of younger people.

How can you be certain you are getting enough folic acid to be safe from anemia? At age 70 or older it seems wise to get additional folic acid in a daily supplement, even if you are eating a very well planned diet which contains all the above nutritious foods in abundance. You tend to engage in less physical activity as you age, so your requirement for food is lowered. Eating any more, you may put on unwanted weight.

This highlights the necessity of daily supplements for older folks. They just can't eat enough every day to supply them with all the vitamins and minerals they may need. And, in the case of folic acid at least, they may not be absorbing much of what they get in food. It is well-known that this is also the case with vitamin B_{12}. Now we have evidence that the same is true of folic acid.

We know, too, that getting quite large amounts of vitamin B_{12} by mouth can result in the absorption of enough of this vitamin for good health. The same is apparently true of folic acid, especially if the folic acid is the synthetic form. It comes as a surprise to health seekers, as it did to the New Jersey physicians, to hear that the synthetic form is better in this case than the natural one which occurs in food. Can Nature have made a mistake, we ask? Not a chance. We have probably made the mistake by not living as we should during our younger years, so that we suffer, later on, from lack of digestive juices and enzymes which are necessary for absorbing all essential food elements.

We don't know everything we need to know as yet about what kind of diet in earlier years will assure us of not entering our later years with defective absorption power. Perhaps it is a natural accompaniment of old age. Perhaps not. In any case, we know now what we can do most conveniently and most wisely to prevent the debilitating illness that ensues when we are deficient in vitamin B_{12} and folic acid.

In the June 10, 1967 issue of the *British Medical Journal*, considerable concern is expressed over the state of old folks in relation to folic acid. An Oxford physician studied the bone marrow and the blood of one hundred men and women over the age of 60 to determine how they stood in regard to folic acid, vitamin B_{12}, iron and vitamin C—all food elements, lack of which is involved in anemias of various sorts. These folks were all hospital patients suffering from a wide range of diseases: heart disease, cancer, fractures, ulcers and so forth.

Thirty-three patients, one third of all, were found to have anemia. Levels of folic acid in the blood were low, as were those of vitamin C. The doctors comment on the fact that these people had been receiving ample supplies of fruit juices rich in vitamin C. But they still showed deficiencies in their blood.

Why were these old folks so short on all these important food elements? The physicians believe it was because of lack of interest in food, lack of appetite, difficulty in swallowing, poverty or immobility. Commenting on these findings, the *British Medical Journal* states that an American survey showed that one-third of all hospital patients at one hospital were deficient in folic acid. In addition, it is known that about one per cent of all old people are deficient in vitamin B_{12}.

CHAPTER 24

Homogenized Milk and Folic Acid

FOR 40 YEARS or more most milk available from commercial sources in our country has been homogenized as well as pasteurized. Pasteurization means heating the milk to a not very high temperature to destroy any harmful germs it may contain. Homogenization means processing the milk to break down the fatty particles so that they are spread uniformly through the milk. Milk that has not been homogenized separates into milk and cream, with the cream rising to the top of the container. In homogenized milk the cream is spread evenly throughout. And this is the kind of milk most of us have been using for the past 40 years or so.

A retired cardiologist from Bridgeport, Connecticut believes that homogenized milk is bad for us. He has assembled considerable evidence that the homogenization process releases an enzyme called *xanthine oxidase* (XO). Dr. Kurt A. Oster believes that the enzyme is absorbed through the intestinal wall, circulates in the blood stream and is deposited in active form in certain circulatory tissues. Here it reacts, he says with a fatty substance in cell membranes to form the initial damage that brings on hardening of the arteries and the possibility of heart attacks.

It is not the milk itself that does the damage, says Dr. Oster. It's the homogenization process which releases the harmful enzyme that we have to eliminate.

In countries where a lot of milk is used—but the milk is not homogenized—there are fewer heart attacks than in countries where milk is homogenized. He uses France and India as countries which use lots of milk that has not been homogenized. On the other hand, people in the United States and Finland drink mostly homogenized milk and have a high incidence of heart attacks.

The French boil their unhomogenized raw milk to sterilize it. Or they boil their homogenized milk. This destroys the enzyme which Dr. Oster worries about. The Finns drink homogenized milk exclusively, as do most Americans.

"I have been around the world twice," said Dr. Oster in an interview reported in *Medical World News* for August 23, 1978, "studying the milk-drinking habits of various peoples, and the same observation emerges repeatedly. Where bovine (cow) milk is homogenized and pasteurized, even if the intake is low, the CAD (heart attack) rate is high. Where milk is merely boiled, or where cow's milk is consumed in miminal amounts, as in India, the (heart attack) rate is low. It is not milk per se, not the milk fat, not the protein, but the *xanthine oxidase* rendered bioavailable by homogenization, that creates the problem."

Asked why women of pre-menopausal age do not have high heart attack rates no matter how much milk they drink, Dr. Oster said that the XO enzyme is activated by the male hormone but inhibited by the female hormone. After menopause this hormone declines in women.

Says Dr. Oster, "Prevention and treatment are attainable, because the goal is to inhibit xanthine oxidase. . . . We looked for a long-term drug, without side effects, that was an XO inhibitor, and found it in folic acid. We employ it in those patients who have antibodies to XO (He means that these patients have shown that their bodies are protesting the presence of this enzyme). Since 1970 we have used folic acid, in 20 milligram tablets, in combination with ascorbic acid (vitamin C) three times a day in a study of 200 patients with atherosclerotic disease (hardening of the arteries) including peripheral disease, angina pectoris or recurrent myocardial infarction. One hundred patients serve as our controls. The average duration of treatment has been four years, with a range of four months to eight years.

"Our preliminary findings, which we view as remarkable, show that in the treated group there has been a significant reduction of recurrent myocardial infarctions (heart attacks), a greater relief of angina and greater healing of leg lesions. . . ."

He tells us that folic acid also serves as a healing agent in the lining of the arteries to repair the damage done by the XO enzyme. He believes that his theory, if adopted nationwide, would stop the crusade to dissuade people from using cheese and eggs which are among our tastiest and most nutritious foods. And it would put an end, he says, to "tampering with good cow's milk."

Dr. Oster's theory is highly controversial—so controversial, in fact, that the Establishment medical journals refuse to publish papers he has written. They are all afraid of controversy, it seems. Don't publish anything that will rock the boat is their general motto. The dairy industry is justifiably upset and, along with many knowledgeable and unbiased scientists, points out that a molecule as large as the XO enzyme could not survive digestion and pass through the intestinal wall unchanged.

Dr. Oster and a colleague at Fairfield University, Dr. Donald J. Ross, have presented evidence that they think justifies their claim. At a December, 1977 meeting of the New York Academy of Sciences, they presented a paper and electron microscope photographs of the process. They also presented evidence taken from volunteers of the presence of the XO enzyme in the blood of volunteers who drank large doses of homogenized milk.

We have known of Dr. Oster's work for some time and have hesitated to bring it to our readers' attention because of gaps in the theory which have not yet been filled in to our satisfaction. Goat milk, for instance, is naturally homogenized. It is recommended specifically for this reason, since many people find it easier to digest than cow's milk. Is the XO enzyme in goat milk? We asked Dr. Oster this in a letter and received no reply.

Then, too, it seems to us that, in order to establish the positive connection between homogenized milk and heart attacks, one would have to know that the same people who have heart attacks are the people who drink homogenized milk. No one has presented any evidence that this is so. The people we know who have had heart attacks were very heavy smokers and/or drinkers. They ate lots and lots of sugar, they drank lots of coffee, they seldom ate breakfast; they were, many of them, grossly overweight; they got no exercise. And most of them never touched a glass of milk, homogenized or not.

The Finns drink a lot of hard liquor. So do Americans. The people in India don't. The French drink mostly wine. For these reasons and many more, it is difficult for us to believe that the homogenization of milk is the only or even the most important cause of hardening of the arteries and heart attacks.

We believe firmly that the best kind of milk to drink is certified raw milk, if you can get it. This has not been pasteurized. It has not been homogenized. It is milk as it comes from the cow. Raw milk sours very quickly. So it seems unlikely that most city dwellers will ever be able to get certified raw milk due to the difficulties of delivering it and selling it before it sours. To compound the problem, various states have regulations governing the sale of raw milk. In certain parts of California, for example, raw milk is available in health food stores. In New York, raw milk is available in health food stores but requires a prescription from a doctor.

However, we repeat, if you can get raw milk which has been certified, that is, tested continually by health authorities to guarantee its purity, *then by all means use that kind of milk.*

If you can't get it—and most of us can't—then there are two things you can do to eliminate the hazard Dr. Oster believes lies in homogenized milk. First, simmer the milk when you get it home at a temperature just below boiling or bring it to a boil. When it is cool put it back in the carton. And back in the refrigerator. The taste will not be changed. The XO enzyme which Dr. Oster thinks is a baddie will be destroyed by the heat.

The second way to overcome the hazards, if any, of homogenized milk is to take folic acid as a supplement. Dr. Oster is giving it to his volunteer group in very large doses. But folic acid also occurs in food, of course. And eating plenty of those foods which contain it can help to make up the amount you get daily. If you use very little milk, homogenized or otherwise, you probably don't need much folic acid to counteract the effects of the XO enzyme.

Foods that are rich in folic acid are these: liver of all kinds contains more folic acid than any other food. Nuts are good sources, also wholegrain cereals and breads. After liver, vegetables are the best sources, especially those dark green leafy ones like spinach, Swiss chard, watercress, asparagus, broccoli, cabbage, chicory. Wheat bran has 100 micrograms per serving which is about one-third as much folic acid as liver has.

Some folic acid may also be manufactured by helpful bacteria in the intestine. However, individuals differ in this respect, for in some intestines the helpful bacteria are scarce and the unhealthful ones predominate. This is true especially in people who have taken antibiotics by mouth, for these drugs destroy "good" bacteria along with the toxic ones. You can help the state of your colon bacteria, generally speaking, by using lots of yogurt or other lactobacillus products which help to re-establish the helpful bacteria. A diet high in fiber also has this effect.

CHAPTER 25

A Relative of Folic Acid Helps in the Fight Against Cancer

IT'S A LONG COMPLICATED STORY, but it seems that at last a perfectly natural substance, which occurs in food along with folic acid, may have broken down some of the prejudices of cancer experts against using anything "natural" to fight cancer. A food substance is being used in treatment of certain bone cancers. It is especially useful for children suffering from bone cancer and was used in the treatment of Senator Edward Kennedy's 12-year-old son.

The substance is the "citrovorum factor". The way in which it helps to treat cancer is very complicated indeed. We'll try to explain it.

The drug *methotrexate* has a chemical formula $C_{20}H_{22}N_{805}$. It is a drug that kills cancer cells by tricking them into believing that it is folic acid, the B vitamin to which it is closely related. The cancer cells stop dividing and multiplying which finally kills them. Cancer cells divide rapidly and wildly so any substance which can stop this proliferation can stop the progress of the cancer. But other body cells also divide and some of them divide quite rapidly, but in a controlled, healthy way. The problem is to work out some way whereby the killer drug will kill only cancer cells and will not harm normal cells.

About 10 years ago, a Pennsylvania physician began to use large doses of the toxic drug to stop cancer, followed by small amounts of another drug called "citrovorum factor" which would perform as an antidote and would protect normal cells from the effects of the cancer drug. The *New York Times* for March 24, 1974, reporting on a speech at an American Cancer Society meeting, says, "Citrovorum factor, also a chemical relative of folic acid, seems to protect normal cells preferentially from the effects of methotrexate, but its precise action is not known."

At the Children's Cancer Research Foundation in Boston, doses of the toxic drug are infused into the blood of children with one kind of deadly bone cancer. Then for about three days the citrovorum factor is administered until the levels of the toxic drug are safe. This treatment is repeated every three weeks for two years.

In *Diseases of Metabolism*, edited by Garfield G. Duncan and published in 1962, the citrovorum factor is discussed at length. It consists of several elements which are closely related to folic acid. Way back in 1948, researchers were looking for some substance in liver which had certain effects like those of folic acid, but was not the B vitamin. They isolated the "citrovorum factor". They showed that slices of liver could change folic acid into citrovorum factor. They showed that this factor was much more active than folic acid in producing certain results in cells.

Other researchers tested this substance in comparison with the folic acid. They found that, in tropical sprue, pernicious anemia, and many other kinds of blood disorders, the citrovorum factor brought relief. They gave the substance in massive amounts and encountered no adverse effects. They found, they say, that the amount needed by individuals might vary greatly. There is no such thing as a "standard dose".

It seems to us that the lesson to be learned here is the same lesson we health seekers preach all the time—the value of natural, whole substances as compared to fragmented, depleted, isolated, concentrated substances. The citrovorum factor is obviously something that accompanies folic acid in food. It should be taken at the same time as folic acid in a natural substance, not a synthetic substance manufactured in a laboratory.

In the experiments reported, folic acid and citrovorum factor were found in liver. Why not give liver? Why not at least see to it that plenty of liver is available in the diets of everybody, so that both essential factors will be present every day to do whatever mysterious things they do in our bodies which scientists are apparently nowhere near fully understanding as yet.

Liver and kidneys are the two best sources of folic acid and, presumably, the citrovorum factor also. Second to them are the dark green leafy vegetables like spinach, watercress, parsley, brussels sprouts, broccoli and cauliflower. A serving of liver contains as much as 380 micrograms of folic acid, wheat bran contains 200 micrograms. Other cereals, nuts and vegetables contain somewhat less.

How many children do you know whose meals contain lots of these foods, that is, two or three servings every day? How can children who live on pizza and coke, potato chips and hot dogs possibly have any store of these valuable nutrients? And why is it so impossible to use facts like these to *prevent* these hideous cancers from ever getting started, rather than trying to piece together a fairly harmless treatment after the damage has been done?

The citrovorum factor accompanies folic acid in food.

Folic acid prevents many of the most deadly symptoms of pernicious anemia—not all of them, but most. Along with vitamin B_{12}, folic acid is our most powerful weapon against pernicious anemia and many other blood disorders. We should see to it that our families have, every day of their lives, plenty of food containing these essential nutrients along with the citrovorum factor which naturally accompanies them in food. Serve liver and dark green leafy vegetables often. Use only wholegrain cereals and breads for the valuable nutrients they contain.

CHAPTER 26

The Effect of Drugs on Folic Acid

IN DETERMINING the necessity for food supplements of any vitamin, every individual must take into account the possibility that drugs being taken are probably destroying some or all of the vitamin. The B vitamin pyridoxine is especially sensitive to many drugs and disappears rapidly from body cells when they are taken. Folic acid is another.

According to the recent book *Drug-Induced Nutritional Deficiencies*, some of the features of deficiency in folic acid which may be induced by various drugs are these: megaloblastic anemia (a serious kind of anemia in which the bone marrow contains defective blood cells.) Also inflammation of the tongue, diarrhea and weight loss. There may also be abnormal pigmentation of the skin, enlargement of the liver and spleen, swollen ankles, heart palpitations, angina pains around the heart, lightheadedness and faintness. Acute deficiency, which would occur if the earlier symptoms were not diagnosed and treated, may bring on severe reactions including an ulcerating tongue, severe diarrhea and ulceration of the intestines.

Those vitamins which are most seriously affected by drugs are pyridoxine, vitamin B_{12} and folic acid. Drugs in 10 major groups are known to affect the absorption of folic acid, to act as antagonists to this vitamin or to increase the turnover or loss of folic acid from the body.

Some of these drugs are *methotrexate* (used in the treatment of cancer; see the previous chapter on cancer); the drug *pyrimethamine* (given to fight malaria), drugs given to prevent convulsions, such as *diphenylhydrantoin, phenobarbital,* and *primidone*. Also the "water pill" or diuretic *triamterene*.

Other drugs which are known to affect the body's supply of folic acid are oral contraceptives (The Pill), the drug *cycloserine,* used to fight tuberculosis, anti-inflammatory drugs such as *salicylazosulfapyridine, aspirin* and *pentamidine*. And an antiinfective drug called *aromatic diamidine*.

Furthermore, says Daphne Roe, author of *Drug-Induced Nutritional Deficiencies,* alcohol—the most commonly used drug of all—affects the absorption and/or utilization of folic acid, along with other vitamins, primarily because it induces a direct toxic effect on the digestive tract, on the blood-forming system and on the liver, so that normal metabolism of these vitamins may be interrupted.

And, to make matters worse, there may be deficiencies of both folic acid and other vitamins, because the depletion of one vitamin affects the metabolism or the requirement for others. For example, when both folic acid and vitamin B_{12} are lacking in the body, there is also a decrease in the amount of vitamin C in the blood.

Then there is the problem of inherited or congenital need for much more folic acid than the average person needs. Dr. Roe tells the story of a 20-year-old mentally defective woman who suffered periodically from the anemia caused by lack of folic acid. When she was given 40 milligrams of the vitamin every day the anemia disappeared. Whenever this dosage was stopped, she became anemic again. Forty milligrams is an astronomically high dosage of this vitamin which is usually given in micrograms which are only one thousandth as large as milligrams.

This kind of anemia which requires large doses of folic acid to control is very rare, says Dr. Roe, but there is evidence, she says, that a much milder anemia caused by lack of absorption, also present at birth, of folic acid may be much commoner and may be responsible for the folic acid deficiency that appears among many women on The Pill.

Folic acid is the critical nutrient required for the synthesis of nucleic acid which is required for cell division. If cells do not divide normally before birth in the unborn baby which is developing rapidly in its mother's womb, defective children are born.

This suggests that the requirement for folic acid is increased during pregnancy to permit normal development of the baby's tissues. Drugs may intervene, says Dr. Roe, and prevent the needed amount of the vitamin from reaching the baby. Drugs that spoil the appetite or drugs that prevent nutrients from passing through the placenta to the unborn baby may decrease its growth, retard the development of its skeleton or possibly the development of its brain.

"While optimal nutrient intake through periods of physiological stress allows a margin of safety to offset variable losses, it is assumed that no intervening factors, such as drug intake, exist which could further elevate nutritional requirements," says Dr. Roe. In other words, when the official daily requirement for folic acid in pregnant women is given, it is assumed that no drugs are being given which would make that requirement higher than the one suggested.

Other circumstances which may cause increased requirement for folic acid are certain diseases in which nutrients are not absorbed normally. Pernicious anemia and alcoholism bring about loss of folic acid, as well as vitamin B_{12} and the B vitamin thiamine (B_1). Sensitivity to the wheat protein gluten causes loss of folic acid. Surgery on parts of the intestinal tract also brings about loss of this B vitamin. Tropical sprue, a disease involving chronic diarrhea, causes loss of folic acid. The antibiotic *neomycin* and the drug *colchicine* also cause this B vitamin to be lost.

There may be greater requirements for folic acid in certain skin diseases such as *psoriasis* and *pityriasis rubra*. The drug *methotrexate* has been used to treat psoriasis. This is known to deplete the body of folic acid. The risk of this medication must be evaluated in the face of reports of folic acid deficiency existing in psoriasis which has not been treated, says Dr. Roe, who says, too, that psoriatic skin conditions do not spread when large doses of folic acid are given.

In 1964 a researcher studied six patients with rheumatoid arthritis who also had the anemia caused by folic acid deficiency. The doctors then studied 46 more arthritis patients who also had deficiency in folic acid. The researchers theorized that the overgrowth of cells in the joints of rheumatic patients may give them an increased demand for folic acid. But Dr. Roe points out that all but three of these arthritics were taking drug combinations which included aspirin. *And aspirin is known to deplete the body of folic acid.*

"Long-term nutrient requirements of patients who have undergone surgery to the gastrointestinal tract may be greatly altered," says Dr. Roe. This is especially true, she says, of post-gastrectomy patients who can become malnourished due to eating so much less food and also due to lack of absorption of folic acid, along with many other nutrients such as iron, vitamin B_{12}, calcium, vitamin D and fats.

Other factors which influence the amount of folic acid the body may have available are income and seasonal availability. Dr. Roe says this is especially applicable to folic acid, because the best source of this vitamin is fresh vegetables. Drug-induced deficiency may be present only during that part of the year when intake of the vitamin is lowest.

Scientists studied the folic acid state of pregnant women who had taken The Pill within six months of becoming pregnant. They found low levels of folic acid in these women during the first three months of pregnancy. The deficiency was found only in the winter in those women who were studied in the winter. Nearly average levels were found in those who were studied in the summer, presumably because they were eating more fresh vegetables at that time.

One hazard of elderly people is the fact that they are the chief users of prescription drugs. A list of long-term maintenance drugs used by people over 65 includes drugs for arthritis, drugs to prevent blood clots and convulsion, heart drugs, blood pressure drugs, drugs to treat diabetes, water pills or diuretics, hormones and drugs to treat tuberculosis. "As previously indicated," says Dr. Roe, "many drugs in these categories are known to be capable of inducing vitamin or mineral deficiencies."

Folic acid blood levels are known to be low in a high percentage of patients with rheumatic arthritis, says Dr. Roe. In 1971 a researcher found that 71 per cent of 51 arthritic patients had low levels of folic acid. All of them were taking aspirin—we presume in large doses which is usual with arthritics. Arthritic patients who were not taking aspirin did not show low levels of folic acid.

Perhaps the most serious side effects due to folic acid deficiency are seen in patients taking the drug *methotrexate*. Dr. Roe describes a number of cases of cancer where this drug was given and folic acid deficiency appeared. In cases of psoriasis where the drug was given Dr. Roe says there should be special concern for patients taking lengthy courses of this drug for psoriasis, for the drug appears to accumulate in the body and hence become more risky as time goes on.

She herself has found that the appearance of abnormal blood cells is "rather common" in people who have been given repeated courses of this drug. She believes, she says, that since psoriasis is not a life-threatening disease, therapy with *methotrexate* should be stopped if indications of folic acid deficiency appear.

We have spoken of various diseases and the effect on nutrients produced by drugs given to combat the diseases. It's frightening to face the fact that what is probably the drug taken most often and most consistently by Americans—aspirin—destroys the body's supply of folic acid. But when you get into the field of alcoholism, the facts laid out by Dr. Roe become horrendous.

She describes a study of nine adult alcoholics who were fed a highly nutritious diet *with large supplements of folic acid*. Two of the volunteers were given additional folic acid supplements of 1,200 micrograms daily plus 30 milligrams of folic acid by injection. Then they were allowed to drink. They all developed bone marrow changes characteristic of megaloblastic anemia in spite of the excellent diet and the additional folic acid.

"Several other studies document the fact," says Dr. Roe, "that high alcohol intake produces changes in the blood that may be due to direct toxic action of the alcohol on the bone marrow." Giving additional folic acid seems to give no protection while the alcohol intake continues. But when the volunteers stopped drinking, the bone marrow became normal again. So there is no doubt that it's the alcohol that does the damage.

"Alcohol has a direct toxic effect on the pancreas," says Dr. Roe, "producing acute pancreatitis and hyperglycemia (high blood sugar) which may be activated by binge drinking. Chronic pancreatitis is common in alcoholics." She goes on to point out that in heavy drinkers liver function is depressed and the stores of vitamins in the liver depleted. . . . "depleted body stores (of folic acid) are found in alcoholics who have been consuming alcohol on a very chronic basis."

It's true, too, that risks from medication causing nutritional deficiency are heightened in the alcoholic. Or in those whose previous alcoholism has depleted their stores of vitamins and minerals. Alcohol is known to deplete the body of these nutrients: folic acid, thiamine, riboflavin, niacin, vitamin C, vitamin B_6, magnesium, zinc and protein. The alcoholic who has become so ill he or she must have medical treatment is likely to lose even more of these precious nutrients if given a drug which destroys one or more of them.

Scientists have known since 1968 that one of the long-term side effects of The Pill is a reduction in folic acid in the blood of women on The Pill. In 1970 a physician reported on seven women who had taken The Pill for at least one and a half years. All developed deficiency in folic acid with anemia. They were all eating nourishing diets which contained enough folic acid. One of the patients was given 240 micrograms of folic acid and showed great improvement in the condition of her blood *within four days*. Four others showed great improvement when they were given 200 micrograms of a folic acid preparation even while they continued to take The Pill. A further experiment, using volunteers who had taken The Pill and others who had not, showed that the ones taking The Pill did not absorb folic acid.

For pages Dr. Roe describes other studies of the relationship between The Pill and folic acid deficiency. Some of these are stories of women who developed extremely serious anemia and serious conditions of the intestinal lining while they were on The Pill. Other studies have shown, naturally enough, that women differ in their response to The Pill, just as they do to other environmental stresses. Some can apparently continue to take it and suffer no deficiency, while others are directly affected, even when they are eating diets that contain enough of this vitamin.

By 1973 it had occurred to somebody in the medical community that serious lack of folic acid in a woman which was caused by The Pill could possibly have very serious consequences for a baby born to her after she stopped taking the contraceptive. Lack of folic acid produces badly damaged newborn offspring in laboratory animals. Dr. Roe says doctors should certainly be testing the folic acid levels in any woman who plans to become pregnant and make certain they are normal *at least six months before she becomes pregnant.* And she should be given folic acid supplements before pregnancy begins.

But, says she, the practical problem remains that there are not enough laboratories capable of assaying the folic acid in blood. So even a conscientious doctor, determined to safeguard the nutritional health of both mother and baby, would probably not be able to find a laboratory which could do the correct testing.

Multiply all these circumstances by the millions of women now taking The Pill, plus the probably large number of obstetricians and general practitioners who do not know of the hazards of folic acid deficiency. Add to this the fact that most pregnant women are taking drugs, some of them as many as 10 or 12. We know the potential for harm in some of these drugs—aspirin, for example. But what about the others? And what about the chances for a defective baby from a woman who has been growing more and more depleted of folic acid and other nutrients before her pregnancy begins, then continues to lose nutrients, due to drugs and inadequate diet, during pregnancy? The chances for disaster boggle the mind.

And these are the circumstances under which critics of the health food movement keep insisting that "eating a well-balanced diet" is all anybody needs to do in order to have perfect nutrition. We can only assume that they have never read any of the above material on the dangers which drugs pose to one's nutritional state, or that they deliberately choose to ignore these facts. And drugs are only one of the hundreds of thousands of environmental dangers which surround us. It may take many many years for our scientists to seek out and identify all these hazards, if, indeed, they ever succeed in doing this.

From our files we find three more somber and ominous notes on The Pill.

March 25, 1969. A woman pathologist from the National Cancer Institute reported at a convention of the American Association for Cancer Research that she had found 100 per cent incidence of cancer in female mice to whom she had given an oral contraceptive. She said that one could not always state that what was true in mice would also hold good for human beings, but it often works out that way. She said also that the longer the drugs are used, the higher the risk of cancer.

April 4, 1969. Medical World News asked a question of its readers: "Will that controversial Sloan-Kettering study—suggesting that more Pill users than diaphragm users may developic carcinoma (cancer) of the cervix—ever see the light of day?" The study was made of more than 35,000 patients at Planned Parenthood clinics. It showed that Pill users had twice the rate of cancer that diaphragm users had. The *News* said that the information was submitted to the *Journal of the American Medical Association* in February, whose editors said they were ready to rush it into print. Now they say that it is "under review."

May 9, 1969. A United Press International report states that a National Cancer Institute researcher has data which possibly link the Pill with breast cancer. Dr. Roy Hertz, chief of reproduction research at the Institute, spoke at a conference on breast cancer. About 67,000 new cases of this kind of cancer are diagnosed every year and 29,000 deaths are expected in 1969. Dr. Hertz said that prolonged use of a mixture of female hormones (the substances used in the contraceptive pill) produced tumors in the breasts of animals. Dr. Hertz, an award-winning cancer researcher, said that his research should be regarded as reflecting a risk in the use of the contraceptive.

"Each physician must evaluate this risk with an appreciation of the many undetermined factors involved and with due regard for the merits of alternative methods available to him and to the patients for whom he is responsible. In view of the serious limitation in our knowledge of these potential long-term effects," he went on, "it is mandatory that further clinical experience be gained under properly controlled conditions of observations and follow-up."

As previously mentioned, pregnant women should be careful about eating grains which contain gluten. Gluten is a protein found in bread flour which causes the bread to rise when it is leavened with yeast. Mixing and kneading the bread dough "develops" the gluten—that is, the pummelling you give your wheat bread dough develops the elastic, gummy quality of the dough which supports the other ingredients, as the yeast releases bubbles of carbon dioxide. So the baked bread loaf is high and light, because of the gluten.

Wheat, oats, rye, buckwheat and barley contain gluten. It is especially abundant in wheat flour, which is the reason why wheat flour is the basis of most modern leavened breads. Corn, rice, millet, soybean and peanut flour do not contain gluten. This is why you cannot make high, light, yeast-leavened bread using only these flours, although you can make various breads of corn, soybean and peanut flour using baking powder. In muffins, cornbread, waffles and so on made this way, no gluten is involved.

Writing in the *Journal of Obstetrics and Gynecology of the British Commonwealth,* Dr. C. R. Whitfield suggested that pregnant women should be careful about eating bread, gravies, spaghetti, cakes, cereals, pancakes, etc., made with the gluten-rich flours. According to Dr. Whitfield, the gluten seems to cause the hair-like villi in the small intestine to atrophy so that they can no longer absorb folic acid. This can cause megaloblastic anemia, he said.

In studying 36 pregnant women with folic acid deficiency and megaloblastic anemia, Dr. Whitfield found that they often experienced a loss of appetite, sore tongue, loss of weight and chronic diarrhea. He reported that, if the condition is not treated, the persistent malabsorption of the B vitamin could cause a deteriorating health problem and eventually might result in intestinal cancer.

Dr. Whitfield reported that a gluten-free diet and folic acid supplements brought relief to most of the women.

Suggested Further Reading

Adams, Ruth, *The Complete Home Guide to All the Vitamins*, Larchmont Books, New York, 1972.

Adams, Ruth, and Frank Murray, *Body, Mind and the B Vitamins*, Larchmont Books, New York, 1972.

Adams, Ruth, and Frank Murray, *Improving Your Health with Vitamin C*, Larchmont Books, New York, 1978.

Adams, Ruth, and Frank Murray, *Improving Your Health with Vitamin E*, Larchmont Books, New York, 1978.

Adams, Ruth, and Frank Murray, *Improving Your Health with Niacin (Vitamin B3)*, Larchmont Books, New York, 1978.

Adams, Ruth, and Frank Murray, *Improving Your Health with Zinc*, Larchmont Books, New York, 1978.

Adams, Ruth, and Frank Murray, *Megavitamin Therapy*, Larchmont Books, New York, 1973.

Adams, Ruth, and Frank Murray, *The Vitamin B6 Book*, Larchmont Books, New York, 1980.

Burton, Benjamin T., *Human Nutrition*, 3rd Ed., McGraw Hill Book Co., New York, 1976.

Cheraskin, E. and W.M. Ringsdorf, Jr. with Arline Brecher, *Psycho-Dietetics*, Stein and Day, Briarcliff Manor, N.Y., 1974.

Davis, Adelle, *Let's Get Well*, Harcourt, Brace and World, New York, 1965.

Roe, Daphne A., *Drug-Induced Nutritional Deficiencies*, The Avi Publishing Co., Inc, Westport, Conn, 1976.

Williams, Roger, *Nutrition Against Disease*, Bantam Books, New York, 1971.

Index

T

U

V

W

Read What the Experts Say About Larchmont Books!

Body, Mind and the B Vitamins

"I feel that "Body, Mind and the B Vitamins" is an excellent, informative book. I recommend everyone buy two copies: one for home and one to give to their physician."—*Harvey M. Ross, M.D., Los Angeles, Calif.*

Program Your Heart for Health

"What is unique about this book is that the tremendous body of fascinating information has been neatly distilled so that the problems and the solutions are quite clear. . . . (This book) will be around for a long time . . . so long as health continues to be the fastest growing failing business in the United States and so long as it is not recognized that the medical problem is not medical but social."—*E. Cheraskin, M.D., D.M.D., Birmingham, Ala.*

"If more people were to read books such as this one and were to institute preventive medical programs early in life, the mortality in heart disease would drop precipitously as well as in our other serious medical problems."—*Irwin Stone, Ph.D., San Jose, Calif.*

"Program Your Heart for Health" contains a wealth of data. I plan to make use of it many times."—*J. Rinse, Ph.D., East Dorset, Vt.*

"This is an important book for your health and well-being."—*Michael Walczak, M.D., Studio City, Calif.*

Read What the Experts Say About Larchmont Books!

The Complete Home Guide to All the Vitamins

"This is a handy book to have at home, for it discusses in clear, simple language just what vitamins are, why we need them, and how they function in the body."—*Sweet 'n Low*

"Want to know what vitamins you need and why? Then this is your cup of tea. A paperback that tells you everything you ever wanted to know about vitamins and maybe were afraid to ask...Read it and reap."—*Herald American and Call Enterprise, Allentown, Pa.*

Minerals: Kill or Cure?

"Written both for professional and non-professional readers, this book offers excellent background for additional discoveries that are inevitable in the next few years..."—*The Total You*

Eating in Eden

"This book contains very valuable information regarding the beneficial effects of eating unrefined foods..."—*Benjamin P. Sandler, M.D., Asheville, N.C.*

"We must be reminded again and again what junk (food) does and how much better we would be if we avoided it. This book serves to do this."—*A. Hoffer, M.D., Ph.D.*

Read What the Experts Say About Larchmont Books!

Megavitamin Therapy

"This book provides a much-needed perspective about the relationship of an important group of medical and psychiatric conditions, all of which seem to have a common causation (the grossly improper American Diet) and the nutritional techniques which have proven to be of great benefit in their management."—*Robert Atkins, M.D., author of "Dr. Atkins' Diet Revolution," New York.*

"This responsible book gathers together an enormous amount of clinical and scientific data and presents it in a clear and documented way which is understandable to the average reader . . . The authors have provided critical information plus references for the acquisition of even more essential knowledge."—*David R. Hawkins, M.D., The North Nassau Mental Health Center, Manhasset, New York.*

Health Foods

"This book (and "Is Low Blood Sugar Making You a Nutritional Cripple") are companion books worth adding to your library. The fact that one of the books is labeled "health foods" is an indication how far our national diet has drifted away from those ordinary foods to which man has adapted over the past million years. . . ."—*A. Hoffer, M.D., Ph.D., The Huxley Newsletter.*

"A sensible, most enlightening review of foods and their special qualities for maintenance of health. . . ."—*The Homeostasis Quarterly.*

"Minerals: Kill or Cure?"

by Ruth Adams and Frank Murray

Foreword by Dr. Harvey M. Ross

378 pages $1.95

In this exceptional book, Adams and Murray tell you all about the minerals and trace minerals: the ones you need everyday for optimum nutrition and the ones that can endanger your life.

In the most complete book on the subject for the layman, you will read complete, in-depth chapters on: Calcium, Phosphorus, Iodine, Iron, Magnesium, Zinc, Sodium, Potassium, Chloride, Copper, Chromium, Cobalt, Manganese, Molybdenum, Selenium, Lithium, Fluoride, Beryllium, Nickel, Cadmium, Vanadium, Mercury, Lead and information about many of the lesser-known trace elements (Antimony, Arsenic, Barium, Bismuth, Boron, Silicon, Silver, Sulfur, Tin, Uranium, Zirconium, etc.)

You will learn hundreds of startling facts about minerals: doctors often diagnose heart attacks by the amount of manganese in the body; chromium, magnesium, manganese and vitamin B6 deficiency are related to diabetes; kelp contains over 26 trace minerals; mercury can kill unborn children; many baby foods contain too much sodium; lead is linked to multiple sclerosis; etc.

"Megavitamin Therapy"

by Ruth Adams and Frank Murray

Foreword by Dr. David Hawkins

Introduction by Dr. Abram Hoffer

280 pages $2.25

This is one of the most exciting books on health and nutrition that you may ever read. It is the first and most complete book on the subject, with over 100,000 copies in print.

There is considerable evidence—and Adams and Murray spell this out in detail in the book—that alcoholism, schizophrenia (a major mental illness), hyperactivity in children and even drug addiction are often the result of a lifelong improper diet. After a person has been eating incorrectly for many years, certain deficiencies and forms of malnutrition begin to appear. One of the causes may also be low blood sugar.

To correct these deficiencies and to return the patient to boundless good health, many physicians and psychiatrists are turning to megavitamin therapy. They do this with a corrective diet and massive doses of certain vitamins. After years of neglect, it may take the body some time to correct itself.

But these disorders can be controlled, as you will learn in this fascinating book. Many case histories tell the story.

Vitamin C, The Powerhouse Vitamin, Conquers More than Just Colds, by Adams and Murray, Foreword by Dr. Frederick R. Klenner, 192 pages, $1.50.

Vitamin E, Wonder Worker of the 70's?, by Adams and Murray, Foreword by Dr. Evan V. Shute, 192 pages, $1.25.

Titles from

THE PREVENTIVE HEALTH LIBRARY

Improving Your Health with Vitamin A, by Adams and Murray, 128 pages, $1.25.

Improving Your Health with Vitamin C, by Adams and Murray, 160 pages, $1.50.

Improving Your Health with Vitamin E, by Adams and Murray, 176 pages, $1.50.

Improving Your Health with Calcium & Phosphorus, by Adams and Murray, 128 pages, $1.25.

Improving Your Health with Niacin (Vitamin B_3), by Adams and Murray, 128 pages, $1.25.

Improving Your Health with Zinc, by Adams and Murray, 128 pages, $1.25.

LARCHMONT BOOKS
6 East 43rd St.
New York, N. Y. 10017
Phone: 212-949-0800